Geriatric Pharmacology

The Principles of Practice & Clinical Recommendations

2nd EDITION

STEVEN ATKINSON, PA-C, MS
National Expert of Geriatric Internal Medicine

Copyright © 2016 by Steven Atkinson

Published by:
PESI Publishing & Media
PESI, Inc
3839 White Ave
Eau Claire, WI 54703

Cover: Amy Rubenzer
Editing: Marietta Whittlesey
Layout: Bookmasters & Amy Rubenzer

ISBN: 9781683730088

Proudly printed in the United States of America

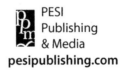

PESI
Publishing
& Media
pesipublishing.com

Dedication

Old age is a window into the past. At this point in one's life, all of the collective memories merge together to create a basket of wisdom. But with age, so too comes the burden of chronic disease. As these life transitions arise, oftentimes feelings of fear or confusion, or even anxiety about the unknown may develop. In times of sickness, our elders will look to our healthcare professionals for guidance. However, geriatric trained healthcare providers are hard to find; their numbers are shrinking. So the guidance older adults seek is confounded by a lack of expertise. If only healthcare professionals firmly understood the dynamics of how medications can harm, as much as they can help, people; particularly the old.

I am a Geriatrician! Which is to say, this book was written as guide for those who seek to understand optimal pharmacotherapy for geriatric adults. I hope to help healthcare professionals understand what it means to prescribe medications, but most importantly, manage a combination of medications in as safe a way as possible. Afterall, "primum non nocere" or "first, do no harm" is a mantra that Geriatricians clearly understand.

I hope this book serves as a way to help healthcare professionals understand that older adults are more than just "older adults." They are unique in every way. From physiology to pathophysiology, from disease states to common medications they get put on. My hope for those who practice medicine is to prudently look at the changes of an aging adult with a keen eye and to understand how medications affect risk! Even in the presence of disease. And especially in the risk of chronic disease.

Moreover, this book is really a compilation of those whom I have centered myself around. People who are brighter and more intellectual, but whose voices I have listened to along my journey, along my collection of memories, in order to create the pages that follow. The most influential are listed below.

Mom and Dad
Thank you for teaching me that with hard work, sacrifice, self-determination, and even failure, anything is attainable.

Professor Les Chatelain
For being my best mentor and THE ONE who constructively taught me how to educate and to do so with a unique style that captures those who I instruct.

Dr. Don Murphy
Despite all of your incredible knowledge, for being the humble person who taught me that connecting with a patient is as valuable, if not more valuable, than what a practioner may actually know.

Dr. Clemencia Rasquinha
For holding my hand along the way, letting go when needed, and most importantly, helping me understand the true art of Geriatric medicine.

Dr. Greg Gahm
For helping me critically think, supporting my decisions on the foundation of evidence, and being a colleague whom I could turn to, no matter what the circumstance.

Dr. Elane Shirar
For always believing in, being supportive of, and caring for EVERYONE! It's an art I'll spend my life learning. My admiration for you goes beyond the words written here.

Mike Lockwood, PA
Thank you for opening my heart to world of Geriatrics and helping me blossom into the practioner I am today.

Ellen Balkema, PharmD
For heightening my interest in, and helping me understand, the critical aspects of Geriatric pharmacology.

Paula Walker, RPh
For working alongside me to care for older adults, with a philosophy that is second to none. Thank you.

Table of Contents

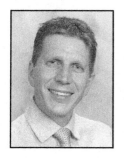

Steven Atkinson is a Board Certified Physician Assistant specializing in Geriatric Internal Medicine. He is adjunct faculty at the University of Utah and has been involved in medicine since the late 1980s. He is a dynamic speaker and lectures on various Geriatric topics nationally. He is a published author and serves on several boards related to geriatric medicine and more importantly, understanding the philosophical grass-roots change needed to care for older adults.

Steven is the Co-Founder and Co-Owner of Twin Cities Physicians which provides "on-site" Geriatric care to older adults. He is also an avid outdoors enthusiast and enjoys running in almost every destination he travels to. He "loves" working with the elderly and considers it his "passion" in life. His positive personality and energy have earned him several local awards in the arena of Geriatric Adult Medicine.

CHAPTER 1

Introduction

Prescribing for the older adult presents unique challenges yet optimizing drug therapy is an essential part of caring for an older person. In the United States, a "Baby Boomer" turns 60 every 8 seconds and by 2030, 20% of the United States population is expected to be 65 years of age or older (Figure 1). In this century, the growth rate of the elderly population has greatly exceeded the growth rate of the population of the country as a whole increasing by a factor of 11 in comparison to the previous century.[1] In fact, the oldest old (persons 85 and older) are projected to be one of the fastest growing parts of the elderly population in the coming years.[2]

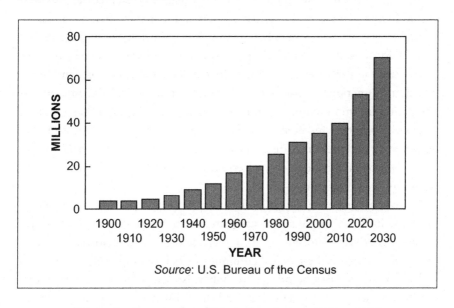

Figure 1: Growth of the Elderly Population, 1900 to 2030

Medications have become the predominant health intervention in today's society to combat the health concerns of the aged. However, as older adults age, there is a strong likelihood of medication errors, adverse drug reactions (ADRs), adverse drug events (ADEs) and drug-drug interactions (DDIs). Common examples include renal failure, GI bleeding, delirium, and falls. It is so significant, that nearly 30% of all geriatric hospitalizations today are the result of an adverse drug event.[3]

The process of prescribing a medication is complex, but the most important question a clinician should be asking when considering using a drug is whether the drug is necessary in a particular patient. From that standpoint, practitioners need to ensure they are choosing the best drug at a dose and schedule that is appropriate for the patient's physiologic status, while monitoring for both efficacy and toxicity, educating the patient about desired effects and potential side effects, and considering when that drug may be discontinued.

Geriatric adults carry numerous comorbidities and, consequently, they are often prescribed multiple medications for these problems. Medication use increases dramatically with age, with more than 75% of Americans older than 60 utilizing two or more prescriptions and 37% using five or more prescriptions.[4] Consequently, the risk of an adverse drug event (ADE) is as universal as the drugs older patients are prescribed.

In weighing the risks and benefits of any medications, medical providers should follow two mantras of geriatric internal medicine: First, do no harm. Second, start low and go slow. These mantras are significant, because age-related changes in physiology and body habitus compound the medical problems encountered in geriatric adults. Since there is such great heterogeneity in the health and functional capacity of older adults, prescribing decisions in this population are more complex and challenging than in any other group of patients in internal medicine. Unlike pediatrics, which for some time has been widely accepted as a distinct entity, geriatrics has yet to achieve this same distinction and therefore, adverse drug events frequently occur due to inappropriate prescribing.

Current evidence suggests that inappropriate prescribing is highly prevalent in older people and is associated with an increased risk of ADEs, increased morbidity, mortality, and an increase in healthcare utilization.[5] This occurrence is due to the medical community's failure to identify older adults as distinct individuals who bring to the table distinct co-factors which increase their risk of drug-drug interactions and drug-disease interactions. With the changing demographics and aging population, inappropriate prescribing in older adults should be considered a global healthcare concern.

Currently, elderly adults utilize approximately 45% of the prescriptions that are written.[6] This number is only expected to increase as our population ages and lives longer. This begs the more important question as to WHY? The answer, "scripts" are driven into our medical system by both patients and physicians, with over 70% of all initial consultations resulting in a prescription.[7] In the minds of healthcare providers and patients alike, the writing of prescriptions often signifies the end of a consultation; it means something has been done. But the misunderstanding in geriatrics is that advice can be as powerful a tool as a prescription itself. Sure, there are patients who describe themselves as being cheated when scripts aren't written and, consequently, prescribers reluctantly give in to their demands. But for the most part, older adults trust their geriatric provider and, if the time is taken to explain why a drug is not being chosen, they are often willing to wait.

Why does the trend of "pill-pushing" pose such a significant risk in geriatrics? First and foremost, there are no studies that can predict the consequences of multiple, simultaneous medications, in any population, let alone one that is already frail and at higher risk of an adverse drug event. Instead, clinicians rely on their experience, instincts, and education about **"a"** drug to make decisions about an array of drugs.

Unfortunately, even the most well-trained providers have difficulty predicting drug-drug interactions (DDIs) in the elderly who frequently need polypharmacy to treat chronic diseases. Second, physiological changes make the elderly more sensitive to medications. Finally, drug-disease interactions tend to be more common in older adults. In order to improve health outcomes, providers need to find a balance between prescribing medically necessary and safe medications and preventing adverse drug events. My hope and desire is that this book will teach you to do that!

To qualify this more distinctly: ***It is possible to arrive at a group of medications that have clear relevance to care, that are scientifically valid, usable, and feasible and does not place the patient at a significant risk!***

CHAPTER 2

Pathophysiological Principles of Aging

Pharmacokinetics, or what the body does to a drug, is affected by four factors: absorption, distribution, metabolism and elimination (ADME). The consequence in older adults is that there are also unique and important changes that affect the rate by which drugs are absorbed, distributed, metabolized or eliminated in the body. Ultimately, these changes synergistically affect the levels of drugs in the blood stream to potentiate drug toxicity.

ABSORPTION

Absorption is defined as the process by which a substance enters the blood circulation. As people age, absorption rates fluctuate. Some physiological alterations that affect absorption include: a decrease in salivation, a decrease in gastric secretion, an increase in gastric pH, a decrease in gastrointestinal blood flow and motility, and a decrease in pancreatic trypsin. But of those pharmacokinetic processes, absorption has the least significant impact on the elderly patient.

Non-physiological factors, on the other hand, do affect absorption. Many older adults take supplements such as multivitamins, calcium, magnesium and iron, all of which can affect the absorption of other prescription medications taken with it. For example, if a patient takes phenytoin (Dilantin®) with calcium, absorption is affected in such a way that it may decrease serum phenytoin levels. If oral levofloxacin (Levaquin®) is given with oral iron (ferrous sulfate or ferrous gluconate), it affects the absorption of levofloxacin and decreases the availability of the antibiotic; i.e., it affects how well the antibiotic works.

Though this is not a given rule, it is a general one: separate supplements, of any kind, by at least 2 hours in any direction from active medications a patient may take; another option would be to hold them altogether during acute phases of illness.

DISTRIBUTION

Distribution is defined as the dispersion or dissemination of substances throughout the fluids and tissues of the body. Unlike absorption, drug distribution changes with age because of physiological changes in body composition in the elderly. Those physiological changes include: a decrease, by up to 20% of lean body weight and total body water, an increase in body fat by up to 35%, and an 8-10% decrease in serum albumin, which is a means by which many drugs are transported through the body. Cardiac output decreases with age and peripheral vascular resistance goes up. In general, plasma drug concentration is inversely related to its volume of distribution (Vd), which in turn, is dependent on the hydrophilic and lipophilic volumes in the body.

Increased fat can affect the Vd for highly lipophilic drugs and consequently may increase the time to elimination of that drug, possibly leading to toxicity. It has long been shown that medications used in surgical anesthesia have an effect in older patients that is related to this physiological increase in body fat. Vecuronium (Norcuron®), pancuronium (Pavulon®), and morphine are some common examples.[8] This explains why it is not uncommon to see delirium long after surgery in older adults and also a reason why propofol has emerged as a better choice since >70% of elimination occurs during distribution phases. The implications of using drugs that are more lipophilic in older adults can be serious, since many of these drugs affect the central nervous system (CNS) and may be delayed in leaving the body.

Decreased body water affects hydrophilic drugs such as digoxin and lithium. With a decrease in body water there is also a decrease in the Vd of hydrophilic drugs. In relationship to lithium, it means there is less circulating lithium available to that individual. Practically speaking, this means that in an older adult, hydrophilic drugs reach steady state quicker and are eliminated more expeditiously compared with lipophilic medications that require more time to reach steady state but are also eliminated at a slower rate.[9]

As lean body weight is reduced as a result of chronic illness or malnutrition, there is also a significant reduction in serum albumin. This may enhance drug effects, because serum levels of an unbound drug may increase. As an example, the fraction of unbound phenytoin (Dilantin®) has been shown to increase 25 to 40% in older patients as a consequence of this principle. This same principle explains why warfarin (Coumadin®) is harder to regulate in patients with reduced lean body weight. There is a similar effect with antipsychotics which thereby increases the potential for drug toxicity. This is particularly relevant when the patient is frail, older or hospitalized.

In addition, drugs are distributed to different places in the body depending on their chemical structure. Those changes affect the amount of drug needed to produce a desired therapeutic outcome. Inappropriately adjusted medications can lead to toxicity or undesired side effects in the elderly.

The most significant example of this is the drug digoxin. Used commonly in heart disease, this drug distributes to the muscle. In a geriatric adult, since lean body mass is reduced and digoxin itself has a very narrow therapeutic range, toxicity may occur since there is less muscle for this drug to bind to. But there are other examples as well, the distribution of antibiotics, carbamazepine, lithium, benzodiazepines, and theophylline are all affected by this principle.

METABOLISM

Metabolism describes how a drug is converted from its parent compound into its daughter metabolites. These metabolites may be pharmacologically active or inactive. In general, overall hepatic metabolism of many drugs through the cytochrome P-450 enzyme system decreases with age. For those drugs with decreased hepatic metabolism, clearance would be reduced and theoretically is reduced by approximately 30 to 40%. This would indicate that maintenance drug doses in the elderly should be decreased by this percentage; however, rates of drug metabolism vary greatly from person to person, and individual titration is required.

HALF LIFE ($T_{1/2}$)

Another concept important in metabolism and eventual elimination (see below) of drugs is known as half-life ($t_{1/2}$). Half-life is defined as the amount of time for a drug to decline by 50% in the serum. It can be expressed in seconds, minutes, hours, or even days. For example, the cardiac medication adenosine (Adenocard®) has a half-life of less than 10 seconds. On the other hand, the cardiac medication amiodorone (Pacerone®) has a half-life of approximately 58 days. Drug handbooks usually have detailed accounts of the half-life of any medication. Pharmacists are also a handy resource when this information is needed. Medications can have one of several fates. They can be eliminated from the body (as discussed earlier), or they can be moved to another body fluid compartment such as the intracellular fluid. The removal of a drug from the plasma is known as clearance and the distribution of the drug in the various body tissues is known as the volume of distribution. Both of these pharmacokinetic parameters are important in determining the half-life of a drug and also represent the transition to the next important concept in geriatric pharmacology: pharmacodynamics.

Since metabolism and excretion of drugs decrease in the elderly, toxicity may develop slowly and sometimes go unrecognized. As a general rule, drugs don't reach steady-state until about 5 half-lives of the drug in question. Steady-state is defined as the level at which drugs rise in the body (blood and tissue) until they plateau and are essentially at the same level in the body at all times.

Since it takes 5 of these half-lives to plateau, toxic effects of medications may be delayed, especially if the half-life is long. As an example, the benzodiazepine diazepam (Valium®) has a half-life up to nearly 96 hours in many elderly patients. Since it takes 5 half-lives before a drug reaches steady-state, signs of toxicity may not appear until 20 days after initial and subsequent ingestion. The equation below elaborates on this.

96 hours × 5 half-lives/24 hrs = 20 days **until steady state**

A significant additional example includes chlordiazepoxide (Librium®). This medication has active metabolites with half-lives up to 200 hours in some cases. Consequently, a medical provider may not see the side effects for up to 1000 hours after the medication is initiated.

200 hours × 5 half-lives = 1000 hours

ELIMINATION

Elimination is the process by which compounds are removed from the body. It is a true measure of how a drug is removed from the body expressed as volume per unit of time. Drug elimination, in older adults, is also reduced because of the reductions in renal blood flow, kidney size, and glomerular filtration that accompany both physiological changes and age-related chronic conditions.

The key pathophysiological changes commonly associated with aging, as discussed above, are summarized in the following table.

Table 2: Key Pathophysiological Changes Commonly Associated with Aging.

Absorption	↓ amount of saliva
	↑ gastric pH
	↓ gastric acid secretion
	↓ gastrointestinal motility
Distribution	↓ hepatic blood flow
	↓ body water
	↑ body fat tissue
	↓ serum albumin levels
	↑ for lipid soluble and ↓ for water soluble drugs
	↓ cardiac output
	↑ peripheral vascular resistance
Metabolic	↓ clearance
	↑ steady state levels
	↑ half lives
	↑ levels of active metabolites
	↓ first pass metabolism due to reduced ↓ blood flow
	↓ microsomal hepatic oxidation
Excretion	↓ in renal size
	↓ in glomerular filtration rate
	↓ tubular secretion
	↓ in tubular reabsorption
	↓ in renal blood flow

CHAPTER 3

Renal Elimination in Older Adults

After age 30, creatinine clearance (CrCl) begins to decrease by an average of 8 mL/min/1.73 m^2/decade (Figure 3.1).

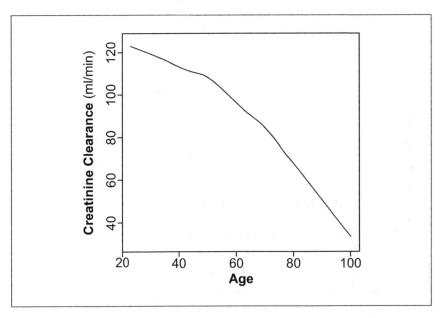

Figure 3.1: Creatinine clearance

However, there is a great degree of variability when it comes to the age-related decrease in renal function. Consequently, using estimated creatinine clearance (Figure 3.2) can result in erroneous calculations about how well the kidney is actually functioning in an older adult. This occurs because muscle mass is reduced in older adults and therefore, less creatinine is produced. By using standard equations that measure creatinine clearance (CrCl), such as Cockcroft-Gault, true kidney function can be underestimated and drug toxicity could result. In fact, the rationale for using the Crockcroft-Gault equation was derived from studies dating back to 1976 when the average age of the population was much less than it is now and geriatric adults weren't as common as they are now.

Better indicators of kidney function in older adults include an estimated glomerular filtration rate (GFR) (Figure 3.3) since decreases in tubular function parallel those seen in glomerular function. But, it is also relevant with any patients with reduced muscle mass, or those who are critically ill, or for those who have cancer. Nephrologists, as specialists in the kidney, nearly always speak in terms of estimated glomerular filtration (eGFR) rates primarily because some studies have indicated that approximately 50% of those with normal creatinine levels have a reduced eGFR.[10]

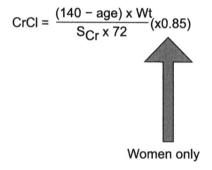

$$CrCl = \frac{(140 - age) \times Wt}{S_{Cr} \times 72}(\times 0.85)$$

Women only

Figure 3.2: Estimated Creatinine Clearance (CrCl)

This concept is often poorly understood even by the most knowledgeable practitioners. To elaborate, to use serum creatinine alone is not an accurate index of kidney function. The National Kidney Foundation asserts the use of the serum creatinine levels as an index of GFR rests on three important assumptions:

(1) creatinine is an ideal filtration marker whose clearance approximates GFR

(2) creatinine excretion rate is constant among individuals and over time; and

(3) measurement of serum creatinine is accurate and reproducible across clinical laboratories.[11] Since these assumptions aren't true in the elderly, eGFR is the tool that should be used to assess near true kidney function.

$$\mathbf{GFR}^{MDRD/IDMS} = 175 \times S_{cr}^{-1.154} \times Age^{-0.203} \times (0.742 \text{ if female}) \times (1.212 \text{ if African American})$$

Figure 3.3: Estimated Glomerular Filtration Rate (eGFR)

The equation for estimated GFR on the other hand, takes serum creatinine (SCr) to an exponential; it also accounts for race where the Cockcroft-Gault equation does not. The following graph (Figure 3.4) demonstrates the relationship between serum creatinine, creatinine clearance, and glomerular filtration rate.

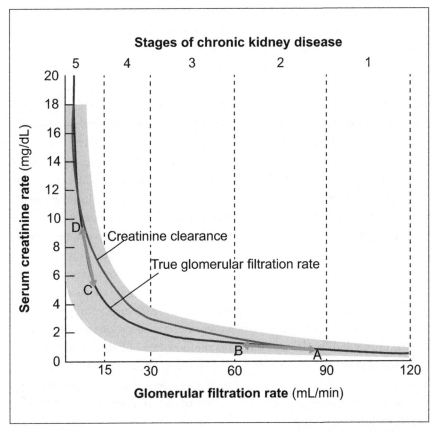

Figure 3.4: Relationship between serum creatinine, CrCl and GFR

As is demonstrated in Figure 3.4, large changes in GFR are reflected by only very small changes in serum creatinine (points A to B). Conversely, minute changes in GFR are reflected by large changes in serum creatinine (points C to D).[12] This phenomenon can cause clinicians to view small changes in creatinine as insignificant, especially in patients with creatinine levels in the normal or near-normal range. In reality, it likely overestimates actual GFR by 10-20%. Understanding figure 3.4 is also useful because it demonstrates that when GFR is ≥ 60mL/min/1.73 m^2 there are insignificant differences between CrCl and GFR. In other words, Cockcroft-Gault IS useful for a GFR ≥ 60mL/min/1.73 m^2 and much less significant for those with a GFR < 60mL/min/1.73 m^2.

However, since there is an inverse relationship between serum creatinine and GFR, even small changes in serum creatinine, as is seen in Figure 3.4, from say 1.0 to 1.8 mg/dL can, and do, represent large changes in GFR (e.g., 88 to 62 mL/min/1.73 m^2). This is one of the main reasons the National Kidney Foundation created equations specific for eGFR. It is also a reason why international and national organizations now recommend that clinical laboratories report estimated GFR when serum creatinine is ordered.

There is one PEARL to using serum creatinine alone. As a general rule of thumb, for every doubling of serum creatinine (SCr), creatinine clearance decreases by fifty percent (Figure 3.5). For example, if SCr changes from 1.0 - 2.0 mg/dl, kidney function is reduced by 50% whereas a change in SCr from say 4.0 - 6.0 mg/dl is less significant (approximately a 25% reduction) in terms of kidney function. Creatinine-based equations should especially be used with caution for those who either have cirrhosis or those patients who are cachectic. The lower muscle mass, and subsequent lower creatinine excretion rate, especially in Cockcroft-Gault, increase room for significant error.

From there, providers need only plug in the numbers to get an accurate description of kidney function. Additionally, clinicians can download free applications to smart phones that will allow them to have access to eGFR at any time. These estimates are important when they relate to medication dosing as described by chronic kidney disease. More importantly, they will minimize an adverse drug event when prescribing medications to older adults.

Chronic kidney disease (CKD) is the slow loss of kidney function over time and it occurs in every patient and in every adult. The loss of function usually occurs over years—though not always—and is best defined based on the GFR as estimated by the modification of diet in renal disease (MDRD) equation described earlier.

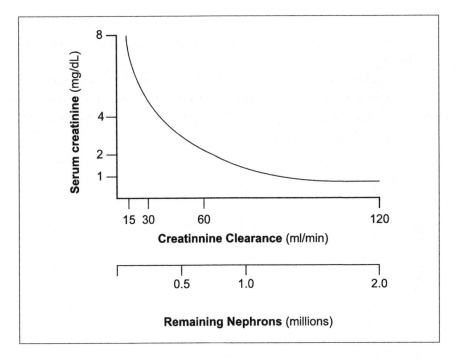

Figure 3.5: Relationship between Serum Creatinine and CrCl

The best models for estimations in glomerular filtration can be found at:

http://www.kidney.org/professionals/tools/index.cfm

The definition of CKD was established by the National Kidney Foundation in 2002 and for practical purposes in geriatrics is defined as a persistent eGFR < 60mL/min/1.73m^2 on two tests at least three months apart. The definition contains two components—kidney damage and duration. This has significant implications in the elderly since a decreased GFR is an <u>independent</u> predictor of adverse outcomes, such as <u>death</u> and cardiovascular disease. As a better clinical indicator, two independent studies showed when GFR was less than 50 mL/min/1.73 m^2 there was a significant increase in mortality.[13,14] Realistically, the progressive nature of kidney disease, as it pertains to the elderly, warrants close monitoring of kidney function. Prudent monitoring of kidney function in 3 to 6-month intervals is probably appropriate, depending on comorbidities. For those who are sicker, more frequent monitoring will be needed as renal function declines. This is especially the case when multiple medications are present or any new medication is added. Additionally, any eGFR that demonstrates CKD in the elderly, requires adjustment in drug dosages for maximizing safety and minimizing mortality.

As can be seen from the graph in Figure 3.6, the risk of death is increased nearly 6-fold as the rate of eGFR drops. This graphic shows the exact reason why the dosage and frequency of medications require a careful and consistent evaluation as older adults age.

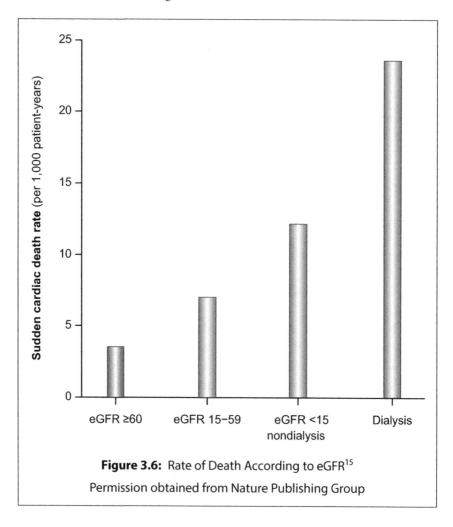

Figure 3.6: Rate of Death According to eGFR[15]
Permission obtained from Nature Publishing Group

Chronic kidney disease is defined by levels or stages (Table 3.1). The stages of CKD are essentially based on measured or estimated GFR. There are five stages, but for practical purposes in the elderly, the decrease in kidney function is essentially insignificant in Stage 1, and only minimally reduced in Stage 2. As was mentioned earlier, in older adults, Stage III CKD or greater indicates impairment which requires medication dosing adjustments and considerations of the potential for harm when introducing medications.

Table 3.1 Stages of Chronic Kidney Disease

Stage	GFR (mL/min/1.73 m^2)	Description
I	≥90	Normal kidney function but structural abnormalities suggest kidney disease
II	60-89	Mildly reduced kidney function
III	30-59	Moderately reduced kidney function
IV	15-29	Severely reduced kidney function
V	<15	End-Stage Renal Disease (ESRD)

With that understanding, a medical provider should make reasonable considerations about dose adjustments of medications, but more importantly, realize the use of serum creatinine alone is a very poor tool to measure overall kidney function. Table 3.2 is a clear demonstration how serum creatinine underestimates glomerular filtration and thereby may lead to risky practicing techniques that could cause harm.

Table 3.2 Comparison of SCr and Egfr

A Very Different eGFR for the same Serum Creatinine (SCr)			
	22 year-old African-American Man	60 year-old Caucasian Man	79 year-old Caucasian Woman
Serum creatinine	1.2mg/dL	1.2mg/dL	1.2 mg/dL
GFR (MDRD equation)	98 mL/min/ 1.73 m^2	65 mL/min/ 1.73 m^2	46 mL/min/ 1.73 m^2
Classification of CKD	Normal GFR	Stage II CKD	Stage III CKD

As is observed, this table demonstrates the significant degree to which kidney function can be reduced when looking at the whole picture rather than creatinine alone. Age is, and can be, a risk factor for declining renal function.

However, Table 3.3 takes this a step further by comparing creatinine clearance with glomerular filtration rate. It is meant to demonstrate risks associated with using CrCl over what should be considered the gold-standard: GFR.

Table 3.3 Comparison of CrCl and GFR

Age (years)	Serum Cr (mg/dL)	Creatinine Clearance (mL/min)	Glomerular Filtration Rate (mL/min/1.73 m^2)
30	1.1	64	62
50	1.1	52	56
70	1.1	41	49
85	1.1	32	47

As can clearly be seen in Table 3.3, using CrCl could markedly underestimate how the kidney is actually functioning (especially as the patient ages). In the patient used in this example, CrCl remains well preserved even up to 85 years of age. But as a comparison, eGFR is at stage III CKD as early as age fifty in this same patient. Even more alarming, by age 70, this patient's eGFR suggests an increased risk of death despite a CrCl that is fairly well preserved.[16,17]

Simply put, an understanding of renal aging by itself is associated with alterations in renal morphology and a decline in renal function. Now add comorbidities to the picture, such as diabetes mellitus, hypertension, drug toxicity, congestive heart failure, etc. and significant risk is brought to the table. Being an astute practitioner minimizes this risk substantially.

CHAPTER 4

Age–Related Changes in Pharmacodynamics and Pharmacokinetics

Pharmacodynamics is the study of the biochemical and physiological effects of drugs on the body. Pharmacodynamics, along with pharmacokinetics (what the body does to a drug), explains the mechanisms of drug action and the relationship between drug concentration and an individual's response to that drug. In older adults, the effects of similar drug concentrations (sensitivity) may be greater or smaller than those in younger people. As an example, older adults receiving morphine sulfate are more prone to an acute analgesic effect; i.e., they are more prone to sedation with the same dose of morphine sulfate than a younger adult. Albuterol on the other hand, has a less potent effect on older adults than it does younger adults. As a general rule, expect sensitivities to most drugs in the elderly to be enhanced or heightened.

The main contributors to altered pharmacokinetics include a reduction in liver size of nearly 25-35%[18] and a decrease in hepatic blood flow; the result of which is reduced drug clearance. Changes in hepatic size and blood flow also contribute to reduced first pass metabolism by the liver. Other factors, as described in Chapter 2, also affect pharmacokinetics.

Pharmacodynamics, on the other hand, is concerned not only with the therapeutic effects of drugs, but also their toxic and adverse effects as well. From a physiological standpoint, pharmacodynamics depends on the concentration of the drug at the receptor site, the response at that receptor site, and post-receptor events that occur. Consequently, the effect of a drug is determined by that drug's binding with its receptor. Examples would include receptors

19

present on neurons in the central nervous system (i.e., opiate receptors) to depress pain sensation, or cardiac muscle to affect the intensity of contraction (i.e., digoxin), or even receptors within an organism foreign to the body (i.e., bacteria or parasite) to disrupt maintenance of that organism.

All these aspects of pharmacodynamics may be affected by aging. As was discussed above, the study of these changes is complicated by reduced drug clearance in the elderly. In essence, with the same drug concentration, at the same site of action, significant differences in the response to several drugs can be observed in older patients as compared to younger patients.

The table below lists some examples of this:

Table 4: Drug Effects in the Elderly

Drug Class	Pharmacodynamic Effects	Clinical Recommendations
Anticoagulants – specifically warfarin	Increased sensitivity	Initiate lower than recommended doses in elderly and follow INRs more closely initially
Antipscyhotics	Increased sensitivity	Be aware of increased risk of falls
β-Adrenergic Blockers	β-receptors less responsive	May require greater β-blocker doses to have same effect
Benzodiazepines	Increased sensitivity	Avoid or use the lowest tolerable dose
Diuretics	Increased sensitivity	Monitor blood pressure and electrolytes
Fluoroquinolones	Increased sensitivity	Monitor for increased CNS effects (delirium) and nephrotoxicity

In general, pharmacodynamics is of particular importance when medicines, like those described above, pose a risk of falls and fractures and delirium; these are lethal for older adults. Falls are the leading cause of injury death for those 65 and older,[19] and delirium has a 10-fold increased risk of death associated with it.[20] This is explained in more detail in Chapters 5-8.

Another concern is that the efficacy of some drugs can decrease with continued use. This is referred to as tolerance. Tolerance may be caused by both pharmacodynamic and pharmacokinetic factors. Pharmacodynamic tolerance occurs when the same concentration at a particular receptor site results in a reduced effect with repeated exposure; a concept known as tachyphylaxis. Probably the best example of drug tolerance or tachyphylaxis is the use of opioids in the management of chronic pain. It is not uncommon to find patients requiring increased doses of the same opioid over time. An option may be to switch from one opioid to another where the pharmacodynamic and pharmacokinetic properties of the new opioid may differ. Subsequently, the patient may have a better response to the new opioid.

One way of evaluating this is by therapeutic drug monitoring. Therapeutic drug monitoring is defined as the use of assay procedures for determining the drug concentrations in plasma. With that information, an interpretation can be made regarding safety and efficacy. Used in combination with observations of the drug's expected clinical effects, such as might be ascertained by conducting a good physical exam, it can provide an approach to optimal drug therapy. But this is only valuable when:

(**1**) A good correlation exists between the drug's plasma concentration and the expected pharmacologic response.

(**2**) There is little variation in plasma drug concentrations from a given dose.

(**3**) The drug has a narrow therapeutic index rather than no well-defined therapeutic concentration range.

(**4**) There are no significant consequences associated with too high or too low levels.

Here's an example of how the above might be applied.

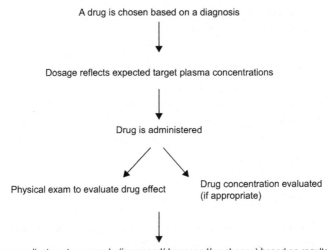

A drug is chosen based on a diagnosis

↓

Dosage reflects expected target plasma concentrations

↓

Drug is administered

Physical exam to evaluate drug effect   Drug concentration evaluated (if appropriate)

↓

Dosage adjustments are made (increased/decreased/no change) based on results

The example used above explains why the dosage adjustment dilemma and age-related adverse drug reactions have brought wide attention to pharmacodynamics. Optimal pharmacotherapy in the elderly is a delicate balance between overprescribing and underprescribing. Realistically, it's a balance between choosing the correct drug, at the correct dose, that targets the appropriate condition but MOST importantly, asking, is the drug really necessary for the patient? The word "necessary" should really mandate the consideration of non-pharmacological approaches to treatment **first**, then assess whether a pharmacological approach is indeed necessary. An unknown, but highly intellectual, source is quoted as saying: *avoid a pill for every ill.*

Figure 4.1 lists inappropriate or overprescribed medications in the elderly, but just as there are those medications that are inappropriately prescribed, there are, as well, those medications that tend to be underprescribed.

COMMON INAPPROPRIATE / OVERPRESCRIBED AND UNDER PRESCRIBED MEDICATIONS / CLASSES IN THE ELDERLY

INAPPROPRIATE / OVERPRESCRIBED

- anticholinergic agents
- urinary and GI antispasmodics
- antipsychotics
- benzodiazepines
- digoxin for diastolic dysfunction
- dipyridamole
- H_2 receptor antagonists
- laxatives and stool softeners
- opioids
- NSAIDs (non-steroidal anti-inflammatory drugs)
- PPIs (proton-pump inhibitors)
- sedating antihistamines (H_1 receptor antagonists; e.g., diphenhydramine)
- TCAs (triclyclic antidepressants)
- vitamins and minerals

UNDERPRESCRIBED

- ACE inhibitors for patients with diabetes and proteinuria
- ARBs (angiotensin-receptor blockers)

- anticoagulants
- antihypertensive and diuretics as evidenced by uncontrolled hypertension
- B-blockers for patients after MI or with heart failure
- bronchodilators
- opioids
- PPIs or misoprostol for GI protection with NSAID use
- statins – *can be overprescribed in some adults*
- vitamin D and calcium for patients with or at risk of osteoporosis

Figure 4.1: Common Inappropriate / Overprescribed and Underprescribed Medications/Classes in the Elderly[21]

It's important to remember this list serves as a guideline, not a rule. You may have even noticed opioids exist in both lists. As is noted above, limiting medications to avoid overprescribing can result in underprescribing. The harm that comes from underprescribing is as serious as that from overprescribing. However, it must be mentioned that underprescribing is based on guidelines that address individual disease entities. For example: a patient with a myocardial infarction and a history of diabetes would typically be prescribed a beta-blocker, an ACE inhibitor, a "baby" aspirin, a statin, and a medication or two to control blood sugar. In this context, clinicians may make informed decisions to "underprescribe" in order to facilitate compliance with some medications over others, or to limit drug interactions. In some cases, clinicians may prioritize quality of life over preventive therapies.

However, underprescribing also occurs from the assumption that older adults will not benefit from medications whose intent is primary or secondary prevention, or from aggressive management of chronic conditions like hypertension, diabetes, COPD, osteoporosis or congestive heart failure. In one study, underuse of medications was found to be as high as sixty-four percent.[22]

When it comes to our frail elderly it's not medication reduction that's necessarily of more value, it's better medication justifiability. The most appropriate medication regimen is not the smallest number of pills, it's not even the safest pills on the market, it's the smallest number of medications that will help the patient achieve a satisfactory level of activities of daily living (ADLs). This is one reason why some people refer to medicine as *an art*; it's a balance of enhancing quality of life and safety while optimizing quantity of life.

CHAPTER 5

Adverse Drug Events and Polypharmacy

Adverse drug events (ADEs) are defined as any injury resulting from drug therapy. It is the most serious consequence of inappropriate prescribing. Common ADEs are oversedation, falls and fractures, bleeding, hallucinations and confusion. More than 95% of ADEs that occur in the elderly are considered predictable and approximately 50% are considered preventable.[23] One study suggested that there were 2 million serious adverse drug events (ADEs) annually[24] while recent studies show us that annually, ADEs account for *over* 100,000 deaths.[25] If ADEs were ranked as a disease, it would be between the fourth and sixth leading cause of death in the United States.[26] But that's the unfortunate problem; it is not ranked as a disease. Certainly, if medical professionals really understood the risk that adverse drugs events and polypharmacy posed, they would focus more on being good "pill pullers" rather than "pill pushers."

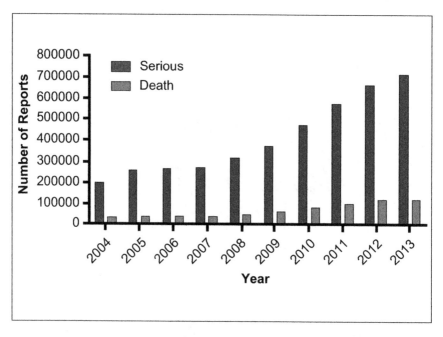

Figure 5.1: The FDA Adverse Reporting System (FAERS) of
Serious Injury and Death (2004-2013)[21]

And, although adverse drug effects can occur in any patient, nearly half
of adverse drug event–related hospitalizations occur in adults aged 80 and
older.[27]

Certain characteristics of the elderly make them more susceptible to
adverse effects. The elderly, for example, often take many more drugs than
their younger counterparts. Consequently, this "polypharmacy" adds to
risk. Additionally, both age-related changes in physiology (Chapter 2) and
the pharmacodynamics and pharmacokinetics of drugs (Chapter 4) increase
the risks of an adverse effect. In fact, the relationship between adverse drug
events and the number of drugs is correlational. Beyond five PRESCRIBED
medications, the occurrence of adverse effects nearly doubles (Figure 5.2).
Once nine prescription medications are reached, there is a 100% risk of an
adverse drug event (Figure 5.2).[28] More recent studies suggest that while
polypharmacy and adverse drug event rates vary, time has still not improved
outcomes as related to ADRs. In one study conducted in an emergency
department setting, polypharmacy increased the risk of ADRs from 13%
to 58% – a 4-fold increase – when medications were increased from two
medications to five. Seven or more medications further increases the risk of
ADRs to 82%.

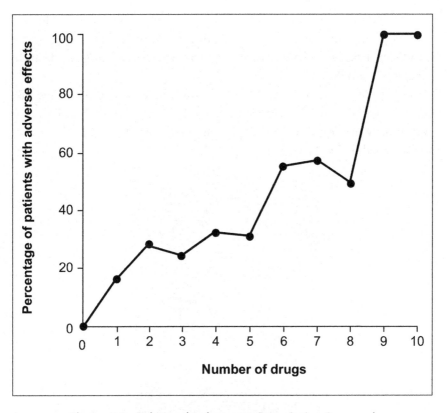

Figure 5.2: Relationship between Prescription Drug and
Adverse Drug Events

However, the belief that the number of medications alone increases risks is absurd. Astute practitioners of medicine should argue that arbitrarily limiting the number of medications a patient takes is counterproductive in populations with multiple comorbidities.

The **primary** reason for ADEs in the elderly is inappropriate prescribing. In fact, up to 30% of hospital admissions in older people are related to adverse drug events that directly relate to inappropriate prescribing.[29]

A drug is inappropriately prescribed if its potential for harm outweighs its potential for benefit. Common examples of inappropriate prescribing include unsuitable drug choices, too high a dose, too frequent dosing, a long duration of therapy, duplicative therapy, failure to consider drug interactions, failure to consider the frequency of chronic kidney disease in the elderly, and incorrect indications. Drugs that are mistakenly continued once an acute condition resolves (as may happen when patients move from one health care setting to another) is another common example of inappropriate prescribing.

A number of drug categories (e.g., antihypertensives, analgesics, anticoagulants, diuretics, hypoglycemic drugs, and psychoactive drugs) pose significant risks for elderly patients and will be discussed in great detail in Chapters 7 and 9.

The Beers Criteria and STOPP/START have cited those drugs that pose the biggest risk to older adults (see Chapter 7 and 8). The Beers list was initially developed in 1991 by a group of 12 clinicians with expertise in geriatrics led by Dr. Mark Beers (Figure 5.3)

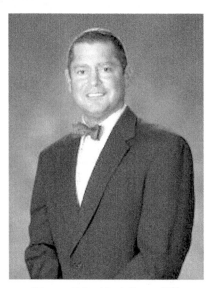

Figure 5.3: Mark Beers MD

The "Beers List" has dominated the international literature since its development in 1991 and has been updated four times since, with the latest revision in 2015. In retrospect, despite criticism of its development, Dr. Mark Beers' criteria served as a dedicated approach to improving administration and safety of drugs in the under-served geriatric adult.

Additionally, the STOPP/START (Screening Tool of Older Persons' Potentially Inappropriate Prescriptions and Screening Tool to Alert Doctors to the Right Treatment) criteria has been validated as another instrument to prevent inappropriate prescribing in older adults (see Chapter 9). STOPP and START are arranged by physiological systems and include reference to drug-drug and drug-disease interactions. Unlike Beers, they address the domains of prescribing *appropriateness* as well as prescribing inappropriateness.

The advantage of both Beers and STOPP/START, is that clinicians are still left to weigh these guidelines and determine the benefits and risks of therapy in each patient, since some patients may actually BENEFIT from drugs listed on the Beers Criteria or on STOPP and START. These tools are guidelines to maximize safety and minimize harm.

Despite the Beer's Criteria and STOPP and START, inappropriate drugs are still being prescribed for the elderly with little consideration to safety. In one survey, as many of 40% of nursing-home residents were using at least one inappropriate drug.[30] In such patients, not only is the risk of hospitalization increased, but there is an increased risk of death as well.[31]

For older adults, medication classes most frequently implicated in an adverse drug event, as noted by hospital visits, are listed in Table 5.1.[32]

Table 5.1: National Estimates of Emergency Hospitalizations for ADEs in Older US Adults (2007-2009)[33]

Most frequent drug class causing ADEs	Percentage (%) of incidence
Hematologic Agents	42
Endocrine Agents	23
Cardiovascular Agents	10
CNS Agents	10
Anti-infective Agents	4
Antineoplastic Agents	3
Others (NSAIDs, Anticholinergics) or Not Known	3
Medications in more than one therapeutic category	5

Of the classes of medications listed above, warfarin (Coumadin®), insulins (Humulin®, Novolin®), oral antiplatelet agents (aspirin, Plavix®) and oral hypoglycemic agents (glyburide) account for more than 65% of **ALL** adverse drug events.[34] Table 5.2 details all of the medications implicated in adverse drug events.

Table 5.2: National Estimates of Emergency Hospitalizations for ADEs in Older US Adults (2007-2009)[35]

Most Commonly Implicated Medications	Annual National Estimate of Hospitalizations (%)	Proportion of Emergency Department Visits Resulting in Hospitalization (%)
Warfarin	33.3	46.2
Insulins	13.9	40.6
Oral Antiplatelets	13.3	41.5
Oral Hypoglycemics	10.7	51.8
Opioid Analgesics	4.8	32.4
Antibiotics	4.2	18.3
Digoxin	3.5	80.5
Antineoplastic Agents	3.3	51.5
Antiadrenergic Agents	2.9	35.7
Renin-Angiotensin Inhibitors	2.9	32.6
Sedative or Hypnotic Agents	2.5	35.2
Anticonvulsants	1.7	40.0
Diuretics	1.1	42.4

In nursing homes, psychoactive medications (antipsychotics, antidepressants, and sedatives/hypnotics) and anticoagulants are the most common medications associated with preventable adverse drug events.[36] It is well known that nursing home residents use more medications than community dwelling adults.[37] One study performed in nursing homes showed that up to 50% of residents use nine or more drugs[38] which contribute to more overall hospitalization and death.

One of the major reasons polypharmacy tends to be higher in nursing homes than in community settings is the clinical conditions nursing home residents bring to the table. In general, they tend to be sicker. Consistent poor health, chronic medical problems and diseases tend to be linked with polypharmacy. Studies indicate that depression, hypertension, anemia, asthma, angina, diverticulosis, osteoarthritis, gout, and diabetes mellitus are more commonly associated with polypharmacy.[39]

Adverse drug events occur at essentially five phases of the medication utilization process: assessment, prescribing, dispensing, administration, and monitoring.[40] Each of these phases provides an opportunity for healthcare providers to create a problem. On the other hand, it's also the place to target potential ADEs so that they don't occur in the first place.

As an example, when older adults are prescribed drugs for minor symptoms, practitioners should consider whether a non-pharmacological approach could be considered. If practitioners decide pharmacological treatment is warranted (e.g., analgesics, H_2 blockers, hypnotics, or laxatives), then consider writing time-limited prescriptions; e.g., Duonebs 4x/day for one week then discontinue.

Solving the problem of inappropriate prescribing in the elderly isn't just about considering a short list of drugs and noting drug categories of concern. Inappropriate prescribing is remedied by a constant review of a patient's entire drug regimen, evaluating benefit and harm and making sure "new" conditions aren't the result of an adverse drug event. By doing so, clinicians are more likely to avoid overprescribing or the consequence of a "prescribing cascade."

A prescribing cascade occurs when the side effect of a drug is misinterpreted as a sign or symptom of a new disorder. Consequently, a new drug is prescribed to treat that effect. This is heightened when the new, unnecessary drug causes additional side effects, which may then be misinterpreted as yet another disorder and treated unnecessarily (Figure 5.3).[41]

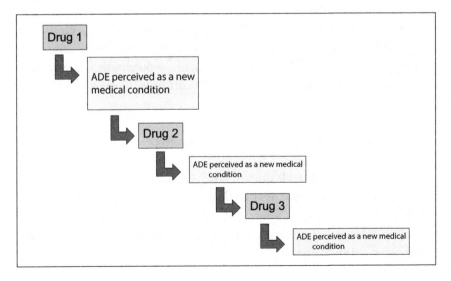

Figure 5.3: The "Prescribing Cascade"

There are many drugs that have adverse effects that resemble symptoms or disorders common in the elderly. Here are several common examples as well as uncommon and overlooked examples:

NSAIDs → HTN → anti-hypertensive therapy initiated

Non-Steroidal Anti-Inflammatory Drugs (NSAIDs) have long been known to cause hypertension (HTN) as well as many other side-effects. Consequently, patients may become hypertensive (HTN). Consequencetly, anti-hypertensive agents are initiated and thus, a prescribing cascade is born.

NSAIDs → blood in stool → H$_2$ blocker → delirium → haloperidol initiated

Non-Steroidal Anti-Inflammatory Drugs (NSAIDs) are the most common medicinal cause of GI bleeding. As a consequence of the GI bleeding, H$_2$ blockers are started. H$_2$ blockers have been known to result in delirium as a consequence of their anti-cholinergic properties. The delirium then leads to a very dangerous prescribing cascade, the initiation of haloperidol (Haldol®) to manage the behaviors associated with the delirium.

metoclopramide → Parkinsonism → carbidopa/levodopa initiated → fludrocortisone for orthostatic hypotension

Metoclopramide (Reglan®) has side-effects that mimic Parkinson's disease. Those features can lead to the initiation of carbidopa/levodopa (Sinemet®) which has a side-effect of orthostatic hypotension. The next step in the cascade is the subsequent use of fludrocortisone (Florinef®) to treat the orthostasis.

HCTZ → gout → NSAIDs → antihypertensive initiated

A side-effect of thiazide diuretics such as hydrochlorothiazide (HCTZ) is it can increase serum uric acid levels which can consequently lead to the development of gout. The cascade that follows is the use of NSAIDs to treat the gout. Subsequently, the patient may get hypertensive, leading to the initiation of anti-hypertensives.

SSRIs → hyponatremia → demeclocycline

The rate of SSRI/SNRI-induced hyponatremia ranges between .5-32%.[42] Consequently, demeclocycline may have to be initiated to treat the hyponatremia.

OTC pseudoephedrine → urinary retention → alpha blocker

Over-the-counter (OTC) pseudoephedrine has been associated with urinary retention due to its effect on the prostate. Consequently, an alpha-blocker, which incidentally does the exact opposite of pseudoephedrine, may have to be initiated to treat the retention.

antipsychotic → extra pyramidal side-effects → benztropine

The classes of antipsychotic agents are quite large nowadays but even the newer agents are associated with extrapyramidal side-effects (EPS). Should this occur, it is not uncommon to use benztropine (Cogentin®) as a treatment option leading to a prescribing cascade.

cholinesterases → urinary incontinence → oxybutinin

The classes of medications known as cholinesterases (ChI's) usually include the cognitive enhancers (Aricept®, Razadyne®, Exelon®). A common side-effect of all of these agents is urinary incontinence. Consequently, oxybutynin (Ditropan®) may get initiated to treat the urinary problem.

carbidopa/levodopa → psychosis/delirium/agitation → antipsychotics

Carbidopa/levodopa, better known as Sinemet® has an unfortunate side-effect of delirium or agitation – especially when used in high doses. A common reaction is for providers to reach to antipsychotics in order to treat those behaviors which bring several risky side-effects.

risperidone/haloperidol → parkinsonism → carbidopoa/levodopa

Risperidone (Risperdal®) is a second-generation antipsychotic similar to haloperidol (a first-generation antipsychotic). These two antipsychotics cause more rigidity, tremors and extrapyramidal symptoms (EPS) than others in their class. EPS can be confused for Parkinson's or parkinsonism. Occasionally, carbidopa/levodopa, better known as Sinemet® is started secondary to this side-effect.

As a general rule of thumb, evaluate ANY new symptom and treat it as an adverse drug event before considering starting a "new" medication to treat it. To evaluate and compare med lists from 2 months prior is a methodology medical personnel should be accustomed to. In itself, this will help minimize falling victim to the prescribing cascade.

Here are some additional rules to follow to minimize the risk of a prescribing cascade:

- Assume any new symptoms are drug-related until proven otherwise.
- Monitor patients for signs or symptoms of adverse drug effects.
  - measure drug levels where appropriate
  - monitor laboratory tests where appropriate
- Document the expected response to therapy and discontinue or titrate therapy if this goal isn't achieved.
- Document the risk and benefit of any medicinal therapy, but more importantly, justify whether the drug therapy is medically necessary.

CHAPTER 6

Drug-Drug Interactions

A drug-drug interaction (DDI) is defined as a modification of the effect of a drug when administered with another drug.[43] DDIs are known to increase as the number of medications a patient takes increases, as the age and frailty of the patient increases, as the number of physicians involved in a patient's care increases, and when patients use more than one pharmacy or pharmacy-shops. Common adverse events that occur from DDIs include delirium, hypotension, and acute kidney injury.

As was discussed earlier, drug interactions can take many forms. A relatively common and significant site of DDIs involves the cytochrome P-450 (CYP450) system. The CYP450 system is a large and diverse group of enzymes that "metabolize" drugs as they enter the body; this system accounts for nearly 75% of the total number of metabolic reactions occurring within the body. As is noted by the pie chart below, there are "families" of CYP (usually called substrates) though which drugs are metabolized (Figure 6.1). If one drug is metabolized by one of the same families of CYP450, the net result may be either a net increase ("inhibitor") or decrease ("inducer") in the drug's concentration in the body; this leads to a drug-drug interaction.

This system is easily forgotten even by the most diligent of providers, though it represents a major source of drug-drug interactions in the body.

Since this system affects the metabolic clearance of most the drugs that are taken, it is important to understand it. As was discussed above, if one drug is metabolized by one of the same families of CYP450, the net result may either be an increase or decrease in this drug's concentration.

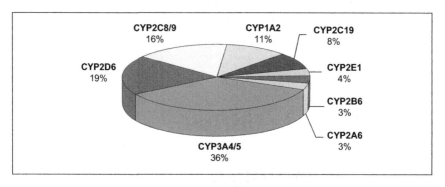

Figure 6.1: "Families" of the CYP450 system

To understand this best, it's necessary to understand the concept of "inhibitors" and "inducers." Inhibitors act to **BLOCK** the metabolic activity of one or more of the CYP450 enzymes. If the metabolic activity of a drug is blocked by another drug, this means the concentration of that drug will subsequently be higher or increase in the body. That is to say, if drug A inhibits the metabolism of drug B, then drug B's concentration level in the blood stream will be higher.

As an example, most clinicians understand when patients use antibiotics with warfarin (Coumadin®), the International Normalized Ratio (INR) will increase and possibly become supratherapeutic. This process occurs as a result of the antibiotic "inhibiting" the metabolism of warfarin; i.e., the warfarin isn't getting metabolized by the body as well because the antibiotic inhibits its ability to get metabolized. This means an inhibitor can result in a clinically significant increase in pharmacologic effects of drugs.

On the other hand, some medications act as inducers. Inducers INCREASE the metabolic activity of one or more of the CYP450 enzymes. If a medication increases the metabolic activity of another medication, this means the drug is "cleared" from the body more rapidly. That is to say, if drug A induces drug B, then drug B's concentration level in the blood stream will be lower. This means, an inducer results in a clinically significant decrease in the pharmacological effect of the drug.

As an example, the drug rifampin (drug A) acts as an inducer of warfarin (drug B). Consequently, if someone was using rifampin and warfarin together, the warfarin would be metabolized at an accelerated rate and accordingly, the patient would require more warfarin to get the same effect i.e., a clinically significant DECREASE in warfarin levels. This patient is likely to require higher doses of warfarin to get to a therapeutic INR as a consequence of this concept of "inducers."

Table 6.1 is meant to illustrate the above. As is seen here, Drug A acts as either an inhibitor or an inducer of Drug B. The consequence is either a clinically significant increase in drug B or a clinically significant decrease in drug B (depending on if it's an inhibitor or inducer).

Table 6.1: Example of Inhibitors and Inducers

	Inhibitor	Inducer
Drug A	Bactrim DS®	rifampin
Drug B	Coumadin®	Coumadin®
Net Effect	Bactrim inhibits coumadin causing INR to increase	Rifampin induces coumadin causing INR to decrease

The list in the pages to follow represents the more common inhibitors and inducers of prescribed medications. To say the least, the list is daunting. Part of the reason for this is the number of drugs that come to market. By November 2015, approximately 39 new molecular entities (NMEs) or drugs were approved by the FDA.[44] Additionally, of the 39 new drugs that were brought to market, as well as those that already exist in the United States, there were 88 "new" FDA-approved uses for drugs.[45] On this basis, it is difficult (nearly impossible) to understand if a drug is either inhibited by or an inducer of other drugs. Simply looking at this list only complicates matters. However, since this is the site of drug-drug interactions, it is recommended that all providers have a firm understanding of common medications whose interactions pose risk to patients.

One way to evaluate for drug-drug interactions is through the newly integrated EHRs (Electronic Health Records) which include "drug-drug calculators" and are now mandated for the highest level of reimbursement in the healthcare system. Other techniques include discussion with pharmacists prior to prescribing. But perhaps the simplest technique is access to applications that nearly everyone can get on smartphone devices. These devices allow providers to "plugin" medications a patient is taking and then cross-reference reactions that may occur when those drugs are taken in combination. It is perhaps one of the safest and quickest ways to minimize drug-drug interactions. Table 6.3 represents resources that providers, and non-providers alike, can use to check for drug-drug interactions.

Table 6.2: The Cytochrome P450 Drug Table (Substrates)

1A2	2B6	2C8	2C9	2C19	2D6	2E1	3A4,5,7
amitriptyline	bupropion[1]	repaglinide	**NSAIDs:**	**PPIs:**	tamoxifen	**Anesthetics/ Analgesia:**	**Macrolides:**
caffeine[2]	cyclophosphamide	sorafenib	diclofenac[1]	esomeprazole	**Beta Blockers:**	acetaminophen	NOT azithromycin
clomipramine	efavirenz[1]	torsemide	ibuprofen	lansoprazole	carvedilol	enflurane	clarithromycin
clozapine	ifosphamide		meloxicam	omeprazole[2]	metoprolol	ethanol	erythromycin[2] (not 3A5)
cyclobenzaprine	ketamine		naproxen	pantoprazole	propafenone	isoflurane	telithromycin
duloxetine	meperidine		piroxicam	**Anti-epileptics:**	timolol	sevoflurane	**Anti-arrhythmics:**
estradiol	methadone		**Oral Hypoglycemic Agents:**	diazepam	**Psychotropics:**	theophylline	quinidine
fluvoxamine	nevirapine		tolbutamide[1]	phenytoin	amitriptyline		**Benzodiazepines:**
haloperidol	propafol		glipizide	amitriptyline	amphetamine		alprazolam
imipramine	selegiline		**Angiotensin II Blockers:**	carisoprodol	aripiprazole		diazepam
mexiletine	sorafenib		losartan	citalopram	atomoxetine		midazolam[1]
nambumetome			irbesartan	cloramphenincol	chlorpheniramine		triazolam[2]
naproxen			**Sulfonylureas:**	**Antidepressants:**	chlorpromazine		**Immune Modulators:**
olanzapine			glyburide	clomipramine	clomipramine		cyclosporine
ondansetron			glibenclamide	imipramine	clonidine		tacrolimus
acetaminophen			glipizide	**Miscellaneous:**	desipramine		**HIV Antivirals:**
propranolol			glimepiride	clopidogrel	dextromethorphan[1]		indinavir
riluzole			tolbutamide	cyclophosphamide	donepezil		nelfinavir
ropivacaine			amitriptyline	indomethacin	duloxetine		ritonavir
theophylline[2]			celecoxib	labetalol	fluoxetine		saquinavir
tizanadin			fluoxetine	nelfinavir	imipramine		**Prokinetic:**
triamterene			fluvastatin	nilutamide	fluvoxamine		cisapride
verapamil				primidone	haloperidol		**Antihistamines:**
warfarin				progesterone	nortriptyline		chlorpheniramine
zileuton				proguanil	paroxetine		**Calcium Channel Blockers:**
zolmitriptan					perphenazine		amlodipine
							diltiazem
							felodipine

FDA preferred[1] and acceptable[2] inhibitors for in vitro experiments.

*A Strong inhibitor is one that causes a > 5-fold increase in the plasma area under the curve (AUC) values or more than 80% decrease in clearance.

*A Moderate inhibitor is one that causes a > 2-fold increase in the plasma AUC values or 50–80 % decrease in clearance.

**A Moderate inhibitor is one that causes a > 2-fold increase in the plasma AUC values or 50–80 % decrease in clearance.

***A Weak inhibitor is one that causes a > 1.25-fold but < 2-fold increase in the plasma AUC values or 20–50% decrease in clearance.

Table 6.2: The Cytochrome P450 Drug Table (Substrates)

1A2	2B6	2C8	2C9	2C19	2D6	2E1	3A4,5,7
			glyburide	propranolol	promethazine		felodipine
			nateglinide	teniposide	risperidone		nifedipine[2]
			phenytoin	warfarin	thioridazine		nisoldipine
			rosiglitazone	voriconazole	venlafaxine		verapamil
			tamoxifen				
			torsemide		**Miscellaneous:**		**HMG CoA Reductase Inhibitors:**
			valproic acid		codeine		atorvastatin
			warfarin[1]		flecainide		cerivastatin
			valproic acid		lidocaine		lovastatin
					metoclopramide		**NOT** pravastatin
					methoxyam phetamine		**NOT** rosuvastatin
					ondanseteron		simvastatin
					oxycodone		
					propafenone		**Steroid derivitives**
					propranolol		estradiol
					tramadol		hydrocortisone
							progesterone
							restosterone[1]
							Miscellaneous:
							alfentanil
							aprepitant
							aripiprazole
							boceprevir
							buspirone
							carbamazepine
							cafergot
							caffeine
							cilostazol
							cocaine
							codeine
							dapsone
							dexamethasone

FDA preferred[1] and acceptable[2] **inhibitors** for in vitro experiments.

*A **Strong inhibitor** is one that causes a > 5-fold increase in the plasma area under the curve (AUC) values or more than 80% decrease in clearance.

A **Moderate inhibitor is one that causes a > 2-fold increase in the plasma AUC values or 50–80 % decrease in clearance.

***A **Weak inhibitor** is one that causes a > 1.25-fold but < 2-fold increase in the plasma AUC values or 20–50% decrease in clearance.

Table 6.2: The Cytochrome P450 Drug Table (Substrates)

1A2	2B6	2C8	2C9	2C19	2D6	2E1	3A4,5,7
							dextromethorphan[2]
							docetaxel
							eplerenone
							fentanyl
							finasteride
							haloperid ol
							imatinib
							irinotecan
							lidocaine
							methadone
							nateglinide
							nevirapine
							ondansetron
							pimozide
							propranolol
							quetiapine
							quinine
							risperidone
							salmeterol
							sildenafil
							sorafenib
							sunitinib
							tamoxifen
							taxol
							telaprevir
							torisel
							trazodone
							vemurafenib
							vincristine
							zaleplon
							ziprasidone
							zolpidem

FDA preferred[1] and acceptable[2] **inhibitors** for in vitro experiments.
*A **Strong inhibitor** is one that causes a > 5-fold increase in the plasma area under the curve (AUC) values or more than 80% decrease in clearance.
A **Moderate inhibitor is one that causes a > 2-fold increase in the plasma AUC values or 50–80 % decrease in clearance.
***A **Weak inhibitor** is one that causes a > 1.25-fold but < 2-fold increase in the plasma AUC values or 20–50% decrease in clearance.

Table 6.2: The Cytochrome P450 Drug Table (Inhibitors)

1A2	2B6	2C8	2C9	2C19	2D6	2E1	3A4,5,7
amiodarone	clopidogrel	anastrozole	amiodarone**	**PPIs:**	abiraterone***	diethyl-dithiocarbamate[2]	amiodarone
atazanavir	ticlopidine[2]	ezetimibe	atazanavir	esomeprazole	amiodarone	disulfiram	amprenavir
cimetidine***	voriconazole	gemfibrozil[2,*]	cimetidine	lansoprazole	asenapine		aprepitant
ciprofloxacin*		glitazones	clopidogrel	omeprazole[2]	bupropion*		atazanavir
citalopram		montelukast[1]	clotrimoxazole	pantoprazole	celecoxib		boceprevir
clarithromycin		nicardipine	contraceptives		chlorpheniramine		chloramphenicol
diltiazem		sulfinpyrazone	delavirdine	**other:**	chloroquine		cimetidine***
efavirenz		trimethoprim[2,*]	disulfiram	chloramphenicol	chlorpromazine		ciprofloxacin
erythromycin			efavirenz	cimetidine	cimetidine***		clarithromycin*
estradiol			fenofibrate	citalopram	cinacalcet*		cyclosporine
fluoroquinolones			fluconazole[2,*]	delavirdine	citalopram		danazol
fluvoxamine*			fluorouracil	efavirenz	clomipramine		delaviridine
interferon			fluoxetine	felbamate	cocaine		diltiazem**
interferon			fluvastatin	felbamate	darifenacin		efavirenz
isoniazid			fluvoxamine[2]	fluconazole	desipramine		erythromycin**
ketoconazole			gemfibrozil	fluoxetine	diphenhydramine		ethinyl estradiol
methoxsalen			imatinib	fluoxetine	doxepin		ezetimibe
methoxsalen			isoniazid	fluvastatin	doxorubicin		fluconazole**
mibefradil			itraconazole	fluvoxamine	duloxetine**		Fluconazole
ticlopidine			ketoconazole	fluvoxamine	escitalopram		Fluoxetine
			leflunomide	indomethacin	febuxostat		fluvoxamine
			lovastatin	indomethacin	fluoxetine*		gestodene
			methoxsalen	isoniazid	fluphenazine		grapefruit juice**
			metronidazole	isoniazid	halofantrine		imatinib
			mexiletine	ketoconazole	haloperidol		indinavir*
			modafinil	ketoconazole	histamine H[1] receptor antagonists		Isoniazid
			nalidixic acid	lansoprazole			itraconazole[1,*]
			norethindrone	modafinil			ketoconazole*

FDA preferred[1] and acceptable[2] **inhibitors** for in vitro experiments.
*A **Strong inhibitor** is one that causes a > 5-fold increase in the plasma area under the curve (AUC) values or more than 80% decrease in clearance.
A **Moderate inhibitor is one that causes a > 2-fold increase in the plasma AUC values or 50–80 % decrease in clearance.
***A **Weak inhibitor** is one that causes a > 1.25-fold but < 2-fold increase in the plasma AUC values or 20–50% decrease in clearance.

Table 6.2: The Cytochrome P450 Drug Table (Inhibitors)

1A2	2B6	2C8	2C9	2C19	2D6	2E1	3A4,5,7
			norfloxacin	modafinil	hydroxychloroquine		methylprednisolone
			omeprazole	omeprazole	hydroxyzine		mibefradil
			paroxetine	oral contraceptives	imatinib		miconazole
			phenylbutazone	oxcarbazepine	levomepromazine		mifepristone
			phenylbutazone	oxcarbazepine	methadone		nefazodone*
			probenicid	probenecid	metoclopramide		nelfinavir*
			sertraline	probenicid	mibefradil		nicardipine
			sulfamethoxazole	ticlodipine	midodrine		norfloxacin
			sulfaphenazole[1]	ticlopidine[2]	moclobemide		ritonavir*
			teniposide	topiramate	paroxetine		saquinavir*
			voriconazole	voriconazole	perphenazine*		suboxone*
			zafirlukast		promethazine		telaprevir
					quinidine[1],*		telithromlycin*
					ranitidine		verapamil[2],***
					ritonavir		voriconazole
					sertraline**		
					terbinafine**		
					ticlopidine		
					tripelennamine		

FDA preferred[1] and acceptable[2] **inhibitors** for in vitro experiments.
* A **Strong inhibitor** is one that causes a > 5-fold increase in the plasma area under the curve (AUC) values or more than 80% decrease in clearance.
** A **Moderate inhibitor** is one that causes a > 2-fold increase in the plasma AUC values or 50–80 % decrease in clearance.
*** A **Weak inhibitor** is one that causes a > 1.25-fold but < 2-fold increase in the plasma AUC values or 20–50% decrease in clearance.

Table 6.2: The Cytochrome P450 Drug Table (Inducers)

1A2	2B6	2C8	2C9	2C19	2D6	2E1	3A4,5,7
broccoli	barbiturates	carbamazepine	aprepitant	carbamazepine	carbamazepine	ethanol	amprenavir
brussel sprouts	carbamazepine	phenytoin	barbiturates	efavirenz	dexamethasone	isoniazid	barbiturates
carbamazepine	efavirenz	rifabutin	carbamazepine	enzalutamide	ethanol	pyrazole	carbamazepine
char-grilled meat	nevirapine	rifampin[1]	enzalutamide	norethindrone	phenobarbital		clotrimazole
clotrimazole	phenobarbital		nevirapine	phenytoin	phenytoin		dexamethasone
insulin	phenobarbital		phenobarbital	prednisone	primidone		efavirenz
methylcholanthrene[1]	phenytoin		primidone	rifampin	rifampin		enzalutamide
modafinil	phenytoin		rifampin	ritonavir			ethosuximide
nafcillin	primidone		secobarbital	St. John's Wort			glucocorticoids
omeprazole[1]	rifampin		St. John's Wort				griseofulvin
phenobarbital	roflumilast		vigabatrin				modafinil
phenytoin							nevirapine
primidone							oxcarbazepine
psoralen							phenobarbital[2]
rifampin							phenytoin[2]
smoking							pioglitazone
tobacco							prednisone
							primidone
							rifabutin
							rifabutin
							rifampin
							rifapentine
							ritonavir
							St. John's Wort
							topiramate
							troglitazone[1]

FDA preferred[1] and acceptable[2] inhibitors for in vitro experiments.

*A **Strong inhibitor** is one that causes a > 5-fold increase in the plasma area under the curve (AUC) values or more than 80% decrease in clearance.

A **Moderate inhibitor is one that causes a > 2-fold increase in the plasma AUC values or 50–80 % decrease in clearance.

***A **Weak inhibitor** is one that causes a > 1.25-fold but < 2-fold increase in the plasma AUC values or 20–50% decrease in clearance.

Table 6.3: Resources to Check for Drug-Drug Interactions

Resources to Evaluate for Drug-Drug Interactions	
http://www.epocrates.com	A FREE or pay drug interaction checker that will display any interactions between your chosen drug(s). Available online and as an application for smart-phone devices.
http://www.drugs.com/drug_interactions.html	A FREE drug interaction checker that will display any interactions between your chosen drug(s) and food. Available online and as an application for smart-phone devices.
http://naturaldatabase.therapeuticresearch.com	A FREE herbal drug interaction checker that will display any interactions between your chosen herbal drugs. Available online and as an application for smart-phone devices. Must register to use.
http://www.lexi.com	A purchasable drug interaction checker that will display any interactions between your chosen drug(s). Available online and as an application for smart-phone devices.

As can also be seen in Table 6.2, the effect of a medication can be influenced by food, beverages, or supplements – nutrient-drug interactions. As an example, grapefruit juice and pomegranate are known to inhibit CYP3A4-mediated metabolism and can inhibit certain medications like some statins. On the other hand, tobacco smoking has been known to induce CYP450 and thereby can have a significant impact on medications like olanzapine (Zyprexa®).

Let's discuss the latter of the two first. The clearance of olanzapine (Zyprexa®) is increased in smokers; i.e., smoking acts as an inducer of olanzapine. In one study, smokers were found to increase the clearance of olanzapine by 98%.[46] The accelerated rate at which olanzapine is cleared by the CYP450 system means that for a patient who smokes, the amount of olanzapine this patient takes would also need to be increased in order to get the same effect.

However, what happens if the patient on olanzapine decides to quit? To elaborate with an example: a patient who smokes 1 pack/day comes into the hospital for acute change in condition; the facility is smoke free. His medication list shows that he takes olanzapine. During his stay he gets more confused for unknown reasons. Why?

Since the patient can no longer smoke, the inducer of the medication olanzapine is <u>no longer</u> present. Consequently, the levels of olanzapine will now rise in the bloodstream since there is no inducer to accelerate its metabolism. This would explain why the patient had an acute change in his condition shortly after the admission. Advice for this patient might be to decrease the amount of olanzapine prior to quitting smoking, then a further decrease after they quit smoking.

More well known drug-food interactions include green veggies, such as spinach or kale. Their high vitamin K levels pose risks for patients who take warfarin or Coumadin. Eating large amounts of these vegetables can counteract the medication's effectiveness.

Salt, found everywhere in the food supply, causes fluid retention and raises blood pressure, rendering medications that treat fluid build-up or hypertension less effective. Alcohol can also have an impact on medications due to the way it can change the liver's ability to metabolize medications.

Even herbs and supplements can interact. St. John's Wort is a potent inducer of liver enzymes, and has been known to reduce the blood level of medications such as digoxin, the cholesterol-lowering medication lovastatin, and even the erectile dysfunction drug sildenafil, more commonly known as the "little blue pill" or Viagra®. Ginseng is an herb that is known to interfere with warfarin. It reduces the effects of warfarin. On the other hand, ginseng can enhance the bleeding effects of heparin, aspirin and nonsteroidal anti-inflammatory drugs such as ibuprofen and naproxen. Even vitamin E, which is found in most OTC supplements, interacts with a blood-thinning medication warfarin to increase the risk of bleeding. Using resources, such as those in Table 6.2, help in making safe drug-drug or drug-nutrient interactions.

Other circumstances of drug-drug interactions occur as a result of an enhanced (not inhibitory) or synergistic effects of medications when taken together rather than interactions with CYP450. Examples of drugs with an enhanced drug effect are listed in Table 6.4 (not listed in order of importance).

ACE inhibitors have long been known for causing hyperkalemia. They may cause hyperkalemia because angiotensin II increases aldosterone release. Since aldosterone is responsible for increasing the excretion of potassium, ACE inhibitors ultimately cause retention of potassium.

The incidence of hyperkalemia can be as high as 9.8% when using ACEs.[47] This should not deter providers from giving these medications since they can be very effective for diseases like congestive heart failure (CHF) and diabetes mellitus (DM) to name a few. In the presence of potassium though, ACE inhibitors can cause hyperkalemia. In the presence of spironolactone (Aldactone®), ACE inhibitors can also result in abnormal serum potassium levels. The combination, albeit very important and even NECESSARY in many disease states, can lead to an enhanced effect of hyperkalemia. As stated earlier, 95% of all ADEs are predictable. The enhanced effects of ACEs and spironolactone on serum potassium are, in fact, predictable. Monitoring renal function frequently (in 3-6 month increments) would likely be sufficient to safely monitor older adults but knowing that the risk exists is, by and far, the best way of minimizing an adverse drug event.

DRUG INTERACTIONS WITH CLINICAL IMPORTANCE IN THE ELDERLY WITH ENHANCED DRUG EFFECTS

Table 6.4: Drugs with Enhanced Drug Effects

Drug A	Drug B	Effect(s)
ACE inhibitors	NSAIDs, spironolactone, potassium	**Hyperkalemia, Renal insufficiency/ARF**
ASA (aspirin)	NSAIDs	**Peptic ulcers**
Benzodiazepine	Antidepressant	**Sedation; Confusion; Falls**
Benzodiazepine	Antipsychotic	**Sedation; Confusion; Falls**
Corticosteroids	NSAIDs, ASA	**Peptic ulcers**
Digoxin	Amiodarone, diltiazem, verapamil	**Increased digoxin effects (arrhythmia)**
Digoxin	Diuretics	**Arrhythmia, Dehydration, Electrolyte imbalance**
Lithium	NSAIDs, thiazide diuretics	**Increased lithium levels**
Phenothiazines (e.g., Compazine®)	Antihistamines and TCAs	**Increased anti-cholinergic effects**

ACE inhibitors in combination with non-steroidal anti-inflammatory drugs (NSAIDs) or ACE inhibitors in the presence of spironolactone as discussed earlier can lead to renal insufficiency, or worse, acute renal failure (ARF). Again, the risk is present and important, but the awareness that these risks exist, decreases the risk of an adverse event.

Aspirin (ASA) with NSAIDs increases the risk of peptic ulcers. Older adults have an increased likelihood of GI hemorrhage than younger adults due to physiological factors. When using these two medications together there is an approximate 7-fold increase in GI bleeding.[48] This is especially concerning given that an estimated 20% of the elderly use NSAIDs in combination with low-dose aspirin.[49]

A commonly overlooked enhanced effect are patients who take benzodiazepines. Any "benzo" (PRN or routinely) in the presence of certain antidepressants and antipsychotics can result in increased sedation and delirium or confusion. The biggest risk for the use of these medications together however, is falls. Any medication, in the elderly, that increases the risk of falls should be avoided unless otherwise necessary.

Corticosteroids have several side-effects, but one of the more important is that they weaken the lining of the stomach. Consequently, there is an increased risk of GI bleeding in patients using corticosteroids. If corticosteroids are used with NSAIDs, the risk of GI hemorrhage is nearly 13-fold higher than with an NSAID alone.[50] Adding ASA to the mix would substantially increase that risk of peptic ulcers and GI bleeding associated with it.

Digoxin taken with either amiodarone, diltiazem or verapamil has been known to increase digoxin's effects. Should a provider see these medications used in combination, it is imperative that digoxin levels be followed quarterly to semi-annually. In general, digoxin has long been known to be risky in older adults. This will be elaborated more in Chapters 7 and 8.

Additionally, digoxin in the presence of diuretics (especially loop diuretics) can lead to either electrolyte imbalances, arrhythmias, or dehydration. It is recommended that any older adult using diuretics in the presence of digoxin be frequently monitored for dehydration and electrolyte imbalances, since they can lead to serious and occasionally lethal arrhythmias.

Lithium, which has a very narrow therapeutic range, should be avoided in the presence of diuretics (ex: furosemide, hydrochlorothiazide, chlorthalidone) as they are known to increase lithium levels. NSAIDs too can have the same effect on lithium levels, so they should be avoided by those patients who take lithium. Consequently, it is rare to see lithium used in geriatric adults.

Phenothiazines (e.g., Compazine®, Phenergan®) when mixed with antihistamines, over-the-counter and prescribed, or tricyclic antidepressants enhance the anticholinergic side-effects of the "thiazine." Anticholinergic agents are best known for their effects on worsening cognition but the acronym "no see, no spit, no see, no sh!&" is another way of remembering the deleterious effects of anticholinergic agents. These effects will be discussed in further detail in chapter seven.

Just as there are medications that can have enhanced drug effects when used in combination with other medications, there are drugs that can have a reduced effect when used in combination with other medications (Table 6.5). This should not be confused with medications that are inducers.

All NSAIDs (including COX-2 inhibitors like Celebrex®) increase the likelihood of elevating a patient's blood pressure. NSAIDs, in any form, are not recommended in geriatric adults but if they are used, clinicians should EXPECT a worsening of blood pressure. This is true even in the presence of

Drug Interactions with Clinical Importance in the Elderly with Reduced Drug Effects

Table 6.5: Drugs with Reduced Drug Effects

Drug A	Drug B	Effect(s)
Antihypertensives (ACE, thiazides, beta-blockers)	NSAIDS	**Reduced effects of Drug A**
Digoxin	Cholestyramine	**Reduced effects of Drug A**
Propranolol	Albuterol	**Reduced effects of Drug A**
Quinolones	Cholestyramine	**Reduced effects of Drug A**
Thyroid	Iron, Cholestyramine, Sevelamer, quinolones, Raloxifene	**Reduced effects of Drug A**

blood pressure medications. Therefore, all anti-hypertensive agents (ACEs, thiazides, beta-blockers) will have a reduced drug effect in the presence of NSAIDs.

Cholestyramine (Questran®) was originally prescribed to reduce cholesterol levels but is rarely used for this since the advent of "statins." Today, you may see this medication used for one of the side-effects it causes: constipation. Questran can be an effective anti-diarrheal medication, but there is one drawback, it can decrease the absorption of other medications it's used with. As a general rule with Questran, avoid administering other medications within one hour of, or 4 hours after, a dose is given. Examples are given in Table 6.5.

Certain beta-blockers (such as propranolol), used for high blood pressure, counteract beta-adrenergic stimulants, such as albuterol, which is used in COPD in many older adults. While both types of drugs target the same cell receptors, one group of medications blocks those receptors, while others stimulate them.

One of the most well-known drug interactions with reduced drug effects in the presence of another drug is thyroid. This effect can be avoided by taking thyroxine approximately 1 hour before or, in some cases, after the other drug, allowing the levothyroxine to get absorbed without interacting with the second drug. Other examples of reduced drug effects are listed in Table 6.5.

Warfarin is another medication that has many drug-drug interactions. Even though warfarin is inhibited or induced by nearly all medications, pharmacodynamic antagonism or synergism may also affect INR levels. Table 6.6 details the effects of other medications in the presence of warfarin.

The majority of drugs increase the anticoagulation effect of warfarin and thereby increase the INR. NSAIDs for example, used with Coumadin, result in a 9-fold increase in the risk of GI bleeding[51] due to its effects on increasing the INR. Aspirin also increases this bleeding risk substantially. But

DRUG INTERACTIONS WITH WARFARIN

Table 6.6: Drug Interactions with Coumadin

Drug A	Effect	INR Effects
Cholestyramine	Reduced anticoagulation effect	**INR decreases**
Barbiturates, carbamazepine, phenytoin*, primidone, rifampin	Reduced anticoagulant effect	**INR decreases**
Amiodarone, cimetidine, ciprofloxacin, clarithromycin, e-mycin, fluconazole, itraconazole, ketoconazole, metronidazole, sulfonamides, thyroxine, gemfibrozil, phenytoin**, salicylates, tamoxifen	Increased anticoagulant effect	**INR increases**
NSAIDs	Increased risk of bleeding	**INR usually increases**
Oral contraceptives (not in Geriatrics) J	Increases risk of blood clots	**N/A**
Vitamin K	Reduced anticoagulation effect	**INR decreases**

*phenytoin reduces anti-coagulation effect by inducing warfarin metabolism
**phenytoin enhances warfarin's effects by pharmacodynamic potentiation of anticoagulation effect

some medications (e.g., most anti-seizure medications) will reduce the effect of the anticoagulant. Carbamazepine (Tegretol®), phenytoin (Dilantin®), primidone (Mysoline®) and many barbiturates (phenobarbitol) will reduce warfarin's anticoagulation effect making it more difficult to get INRs to therapeutic ranges. Warfarin inhibits coagulation by antagonizing the action of vitamin K. Warfarin prevents the recycling of vitamin K and thereby creates a functional vitamin K deficiency. In the presence of an abnormally high INR with bleeding, supplemental vitamin K can overcome the anticoagulant effects of warfarin.

On another note, notice how oral contraceptives increase the risk of blood clots. Oral contraception affects blood clotting by increasing plasma fibrinogen and the activity of coagulation factors; platelet activity is also enhanced as well. These changes create a state of hypercoagulability that increases the risk of blood clots in the veins, such as deep vein thrombosis (DVT). Studies of the oral contraceptives in current use show that the coagulation effects depend on the dosage of estrogen and the type of progestogen used in combination.

TOP TEN DANGEROUS DRUG INTERACTIONS IN LONG-TERM CARE

In March 2001, the American Medical Directors Association (AMDA) and American Society of Consultant Pharmacists (ASCP) summarized the top 10 dangerous drug combinations in long-term care. It should not surprise providers that warfarin interactions made up half the list. The list below describes which medications have the most significant drug-drug interactions followed by a description of the interaction.

- Warfarin — NSAIDs
- Warfarin — Sulfa drugs
- Warfarin — Macrolides
- Warfarin — Quinolones
- Warfarin — Phenytoin
- ACE inhibitors — Potassium supplements
- ACE inhibitors — Spironolactone
- Digoxin — Amiodarone
- Digoxin — Verapamil
- Theophylline — Quinolones (ciprofloxacin, norfloxacin, oflaxacin)

To elaborate:

Warfarin → NSAIDs (doesn't include Celebrex®)
- may increase INR
- increases risk of GI bleeding

Warfarin → Sulfonamides (Bactrim®, Septra®, sulfamethoxazole)
- increases INR increasing risk of bleeding

Warfarin → Macrolides (Biaxin®, erythromycin, Zithromax®)
- increase INR increasing risk of bleeding

Warfarin → Quinolones (Avelox®, Cipro®, Floxin®, Levaquin®, Noroxin®)
- increase INR increasing risk of bleeding

Warfarin → Phenytoin (Dilantin®)
- may increase or decrease INR

ACE inhibitors (Accupril®, Altace®, Capoten®, lisinopril, Lotensin®, Univasc®) **→ Potassium**
- increases risk of hyperkalemia

ACE inhibitors (Accupril®, Altace®, Capoten®, lisinopril, Lotensin®, Univasc®) **→ Aldactone**
- increases risk of hyperkalemia

Digoxin → Amiodorone
- combination may increase digoxin levels leading to toxicity and cardiac side-effects

Digoxin → Verapamil
- combination may increase digoxin levels leading to toxicity
- increases risk of AV block

Theophylline → Quinolones (only Cipro®, Floxin®, Noroxin®)
- combination may increase theophylline levels

Given the recent advent of novel oral anti-coagulants (NOACs), which include medications like apixaban (Eliquis®), dabigatran (Pradaxa®), edoxaban (Savaysa®), rivaroxaban (Xarelto®), it makes sense these medications are now used more frequently than warfarin. There is no doubt NOACs anticoagulate the blood and thereby increase the risk of bleeding, but overall, NOACs had a similar or less serious effect to warfarin on the risk of major bleeding.[52] Major bleeding is defined as intracranial bleeding, clinically overt signs of hemorrhage associated with a drop in hemoglobin of ≥5 g/dL or a ≥15% absolute decrease in hematocrit, or fatal bleeding that directly results in death within 7 days.[53]

Given that safety is paramount with medications that do increase the risk of bleeding, this risk is higher in those older than 75 years of age. In Table 6.7, safety considerations for choosing the correct NOAC are evaluated should one be considered over warfarin.[54]

WARFARIN COMPARED TO THE NOVEL ORAL ANTICOAGULANTS

Table 6.7: Warfarin Compared to the Novel Oral Anticoagulants[52]

Novel Anti-Coagulants	Stroke Prevention in Non-Valvular Atrial-Fibrillation		Treatment of DVT/PE	
	Prevention of Stroke vs Warfarin	Major Bleeding vs Warfarin	Prevention of Recurrent DVT/PE vs Warfarin	Major Bleeding vs Warfarin in DVT/PE
Apixaban	Decreased risk	Decreased risk	Equivalent risk	Decreased risk
Dabigatran	Decreased risk	Equivalent risk	Equivalent risk	Equivalent risk
Edoxaban	Equivalent risk	Decreased risk	Equivalent risk	Decreased risk
Rivaroxaban	Equivalent risk	Equivalent risk	Equivalent risk	Decreased risk

What about drug-drug interactions amongst over-the-counter (OTC) drugs? Table 6.8 describes common reactions that occur with OTC agents. The risks of over-the-counter medications have long been known, but nevertheless commonly occur because older adults are either not informed about the risks of OTC medications, or assume there is little risk because they are OTC medications.

DRUG-DRUG INTERACTIONS OF COMMON OTC DRUGS

Table 6.8: Drug-Drug Interactions of Common OTC Drugs

OTC Drug	Prescription Drug or Class	Adverse Effect
Acetaminophen	Rifampin	Potentiates APAP effects resulting in liver failure
NSAIDs	Methotrexate	Can increase methotrexate levels
Non-steroidal anti-inflammatory (NSAIDs)	Digoxin, beta-blockers, diuretics	Reduces BP lowering effects
NSAIDs	Warfarin	NSAIDs increase blood-thinning effects of blood thinners
Ibuprofen; Naproxen sodium	Lithium	Lithium toxicity
Antihistamines (brompheniramine, chlorpheniramine, dimenhydrinate, diphenhydramine, doxylamine)	Alprazolam, Temazepam	Increased sedation/lethargy
Pseudoephedrine	MAOIs (phenelzine, selegiline, tranylcypromine)	Life-threatening arrhythmia's
Dextromethorphan	SSRIs, MAOIs	Serotonin syndrome
Dextromethorphan	Sedatives	Increased sedation/lethargy

Acetaminophen (Tylenol®) when used with rifampin can potentiate the effects of Tylenol as it's metabolized through the liver, potentiating acetaminophen toxicity and liver failure. If the combination is given, medical personnel should limit dosing of Tylenol to less than the current recommendation of 3000 milligrams. Recommendation: no more than 2 grams.

Any NSAID, when used with methotrexate, has the potential to increase serum methotrexate levels. In addition, any patient using anti-hypertensives should clearly understand that all NSAIDs decrease the blood-pressure lowering effects for any blood pressure medication. Furthermore, NSAIDs when used with warfarin (Coumadin®) can result in supratherapeutic INRs and thereby increase the risks of hemorrhage. Finally, NSAIDs in combination with lithium can potentiate the effects of lithium leading to toxicity; NSAIDs should be avoided in patients using lithium.

A common interaction occurs when patients use benzodiazepines, such as alprazolam or temazepam, with OTC cold remedies. Common antihistamines that can be found in nearly all OTC "cold" products include: brompheniramine, chlorpheniramine, dimenhydrinate, diphenyhydramine, doxylamine. In combination, older adults can become seriously, even lethally over sedated.

Another dangerous, and potentially life-threatening interaction is pseudoephedrine with monoamine oxidase inhibitors (MAOIs). MAOIs are a class of antidepressants usually prescribed by psychiatrists. Besides psychiatrists, neurologists might also prescribe these medications, particularly in patients with Parkinson's disease. A common MAOI used by neurologists is selegiline. Any medical provider who comes across a patient taking an MAOI must pay careful attention to other medications being used with it in order to avoid serious drug-drug interactions that usually result in life-threatening arrhythmias.

Dextromethorphan can also interact dangerously with MAOIs. Any patient taking MAOIs must be informed that dextromethorphan is very dangerous, and potentially lethal, with these medications. Additionally, dextromethorphan is likely to increase sedation when used with any sedative or narcotic agent. Finally, when MAOIs are taken with SSRIs (Lexapro®, Celexa®, Zoloft®), the result can lead to a *serotonin syndrome.*

Serotonin syndrome is a potentially life-threatening drug reaction that causes the body to have too much serotonin in the system. Symptoms can occur within minutes and as late as several hours or days later. Symptoms include:

- Agitation or restlessness
- Nausea, vomiting, diarrhea
- Tachycardia
- Hallucinations
- Hyperthermia
- Loss of coordination
- Overactive reflexes
- Rapid changes and fluctuations in blood pressure
- Seizures

CHAPTER 7

The "Beers List"

As stated earlier, the Beers Criteria was developed as a tool to identify inappropriate drugs or high-risk drugs in the elderly. The criteria are intended for all ambulatory, acute, and institutionalized populations aged 65 and older, with the exception of those patients on hospice and/or palliative care. The figures that follow will list inappropriate drugs in the elderly as originally detailed by Beers and colleagues.[55] The newest update to the Beers Criteria occurred in 2015, and this is the fifth revision to the list since it was released. This latest update includes: new evidence of potentially inappropriate medications in the elderly, grading of each recommendation by the strength and quality of studies to suggest why it was chosen, incorporation of evidence on drug–drug interactions and dose adjustments based on kidney function for select medications and, finally, incorporation of exceptions to the rules if deemed clinically appropriate or necessary.

Although the Beers Criteria is an invaluable tool for prescribing for older patients, one of the major differences between this publication and the publications prior to 2012 is the understanding that the criteria should not substitute for professional judgment or dictate prescribing for any patient when the clinician believes the benefits of the medication(s) outweigh the potential risks. Simply put, the Beers list is not applicable in all circumstances. As was alluded to above, a clinician prescribing for an individual receiving end-of-life or palliative care might determine a medication that may be potentially inappropriate for older adults, is realistically the only and most reasonable choice for that individual.

The 13 panelists concluded that, "If a provider is not able to find an alternative [drug] and chooses to continue to use a drug on this list in an individual patient, [simply noting that] the medication [is] potentially inappropriate can serve as a reminder for close monitoring so that [adverse drug events] ADEs can be incorporated into the electronic health record and prevented or detected early."[56] With that said, the criteria are not meant to be used punitively, but rather, to inform clinical decision making, research and training to improve the quality and safety of prescribing for older adults.

The table below (Table 7.1) describes the quality and strength of the evidence used in the updated version of the Beers Criteria.[57]

DESIGNATIONS OF QUALITY AND STRENGTH OF EVIDENCE

Table 7.1: Designations of Quality and Strength of Evidence

Designation	Description
Quality of Evidence	
High	Evidence includes consistent results from well-designed, well-conducted studies in representative populations that directly assess effects on health outcomes (≥2 consistent, higher-quality randomized controlled trials or multiple, consistent observational studies with no significant methodological flaws showing large effects).
Moderate	Evidence is sufficient to determine risks of adverse outcomes, but the number, quality, size, or consistency of included studies; generalizability to routine practice; or indirect nature of the evidence on health outcomes (≥1 higher-quality trial with >100 participants; ≥2 higher-quality trials with some inconsistency; ≥2 consistent, lower-quality trials; or multiple, consistent observational studies with no significant methodological flaws showing at least moderate effects) limits the strength of the evidence.
Low	Evidence is insufficient to assess harms or risks in health outcomes because of limited number or power of studies, large and unexplained inconsistency between higher-quality studies, important flaws in study design or conduct, gaps in the chain of evidence, or lack of information on important health outcomes.
Strength of Recommendation	
Strong	Benefits clearly outweigh harms, adverse events, and risks, or harms, adverse events, and risks clearly outweigh benefits.
Weak	Benefits may not outweigh harms, adverse events, and risks.
Insufficient	Evidence inadequate to determine net harms, adverse events, and risks.

In previous versions of the Beers list there has been appropriate criticisms about the quality of evidence used to discuss why certain medications "made the list" while others were "left off." Prior to Beers 2012, a doctor prescribing a medication on the list was criticized for using the drug without true evidence to suggest why it made the list. In essence, the list penalized prescribers for their decisions, when in reality, the medication, albeit dangerous, may have been the best choice for that particular patient. Since that time, evidence has been provided to support why the medication made the list.

As noted earlier, this panel consisted of 13 experts in geriatric care and pharmacology who graded and performed a systematic review of each medication that was selected. This author had the fortune to speak with one member of the panel who confirmed that the panel meant the list to be a guide to avoid inappropriate prescribing and NOT as a tool to penalize prescribers. Consequently, the list included not only potentially inappropriate medications, but also classes of medications to avoid in older adults. It also included medications to avoid in older adults with certain syndromes and/ or diseases (see Chapter 8). New to the 2015 Beers criteria are potentially clinically important drug–drug interactions (Chapter 8) and medications to avoid or adjust the dosage based on the individual's kidney function (Chapter 8).

The following Figures (Tables 7.2, 7.4-7.7, 7.10-7.14) detail ALL of the medications included in the Beers criteria.[58] However, the discussions that follow each table will include only medications that practitioners may commonly see.

First generation antihistamines are commonly found over-the-counter nowadays. Common examples include diphenhydramine (Benadryl®), chlorpheniramine (Chlor-Trimeton®) and doxylamine (Unisom®). Other first generation antihistamines are prescribed: cyproheptadine (Periactin®), hydroxyzine (Atarax®), promethazine (Phenergan®).

All first-generation antihistamines are highly anticholinergic with side-effects that can be remembered with the phrase "no see, no spit, no pee, no sh!&." More appropriately, however, anticholinergic agents are infamous for causing "anti-SLUD." This acronym includes the main features of anticholinergic agents: anti-salivation, anti-lacrimation, anti-urination and anti-defecation. Figure 7.3 shows all of the dangerous and serious side-effects of anticholinergic agents. Benadryl® is one of those agents that makes the top ten list of medications to avoid in geriatrics (see Chapter 10).

Table 7.2: First Generation Antihistamines

Organ System or Therapeutic Category or Drug	Rationale	Recommendation	Quality/ Strength
First-generation antihistamines			
• Brompheniramine • Carbinoxamine • Chlorpheniramine • Clemastine • Cyproheptadine • Dexbrompheniramine • Dexchlorpheniramine • Dimenhydrinate • Diphenhydramine (oral) • Doxylamine • Hydroxyzine • Meclizine • Promethazine • Triprolidine	Highly anticholinergic; clearance reduced with advanced age, and tolerance develops when used as hypnotic; greater risk of confusion, dry mouth, constipation, and other anticholinergic effects and toxicity. Use of diphenhydramine in special situations such as acute treatment of severe allergic reaction may be appropriate.	**Avoid**	Moderate/ Strong

Table 7.3: Symptoms of Anticholinergic Drugs

Physical Symptoms	Cognitive Symptoms
Blurred vision	Confusion / clouding of consciousness
Hot, dry skin / dehydration	Memory impairment
Dry mouth	Visual hallucinations
Shortness of breath	Sensory illusions
Dilated pupils	Disturbance in sleep-wake cycle
Increased heart rate	Disorientation, especially to time and place
Increased / decreased psychomotor activity	Incoherent speech
Anorexia	Anxiety, agitation, excitement
Urinary Retention	

As can clearly be seen, both the physical and cognitive side-effects of these agents are quite severe and explain, quite simply, why these agents should be avoided when feasible.

Patients who may be taking anticholinergic drugs (see Tables 7.1-7.3), can appear "demented" when in actuality it's a drug effect; remove the drug and the patient may demonstrate memory improvement. It is also important to understand that cholinergic drugs do the exact opposite of anticholinergics and that when taken together the cholinergic effects are negated. In other words, the cholinergic drugs – donepezil (Aricept®), rivastigmine (Exelon®) and galantamine (Razadyne®) – which are touted to improve memory in those with dementia, are ineffective in the presence of any anticholinergic agent.

Any anticholinergic drug also has reduced clearance in those with advanced age which poses a significant risk of both delirium and renal failure. And, when these medications are used as sleep aids, tolerance can occur requiring higher and higher doses to achieve the same effect which eventually risks toxicity. On the other hand, Benadryl® (diphenhydramine) can and perhaps even should be used in situations such as acute treatment of severe allergic reactions.

The recommendation overall, as described in the Beers criteria, is to generally avoid first-generation antihistamines in geriatric adults. The quality of evidence to support this recommendation is "moderate" while the strength of the recommendation is strong.

Table 7.4: Antiparkinsonian Agents

Organ System or Therapeutic Category or Drug	Rationale	Recommendation	Quality/ Strength
Benztropine (oral) Trihexyphenidyl	Not recommended for prevention of EPS with antipsychotics; more-effective agents available for treatment of Parkinson's.	**Avoid**	Moderate/ Strong

Other anticholinergic agents are antiparkinson's agents (Table 7.4). Two of the agents that made the Beers Criteria are oral benztropine (Cogentin®) and trihexyphenidyl (Artane®). Both are used for parkinsonisms or extrapyramidal reactions that may occur with drugs used to control features associated with Parkinson's disease or parkinsonism. Nowadays, there are generally more effective agents than the ones described here; therefore, the recommendation in geriatrics is to avoid them. The quality of evidence is moderate, and the strength of that recommendation is strong.

ANTICHOLINERGICS (ANTISPASMODICS)

Table 7.5: Antispasmodics

Organ System or Therapeutic Category or Drug	Rationale	Recommendation	Quality/ Strength
• Atropine (excludes ophthalmic) • Belladonna alkaloids • Trihexyphenidyl • Clidinium-chlordiazepoxide • Dicyclomine • Hyoscyamine • Propantheline • Scopolamine	Highly anticholinergic, uncertain effectiveness.	**Avoid**	Moderate/Strong

Additional anticholinergic agents include drugs used for GI tract spasms; a class of medications called antispasmodics (Table 7.5). Common examples include: atropine (excludes ophthalmic), belladonna alkaloids (Donnatal®), dicyclomine (Bentyl®), hyoscyamine (Levsin®) and scopolamine (Scopace®). These medications tend to be very anticholinergic but have uncertain effectiveness. The general recommendation in geriatrics is to avoid them; however, there may be some clinical benefit short-term for those patients in palliative or hospice care and they could be considered in such a situation. The quality of evidence that exists for the antispasmodics is moderate while the strength of the recommendation is strong.

Table 7.6: Antithrombotics

Organ System or Therapeutic Category or Drug	Rationale	Recommendation	Quality/ Strength
Dipyridamole, oral short-acting (does not apply to the extended release combination with aspirin)	May cause orthostatic hypotension; more-effective alternatives available; IV form acceptable for use in cardiac stress test.	**Avoid**	Moderate/ Strong
Ticlopidine	Safer effective alternatives available.	**Avoid**	Moderate/ Strong

Two antithrombotics have been placed on the Beers list (Table 7.6). Dipyridamole (Persantine®) in the oral short-acting form was placed on the list as it has been known to cause orthostatic hypotension. It is important to note the IV form is still acceptable for use in patients undergoing a cardiac stress test as well as the long-acting oral formulation. Ticlopidine (Ticlid®) is the second agent. The quality of evidence to support the recommendations for both of these medications is moderate while the strength behind the recommendation is strong.

Table 7.7: Anti-infective

Organ System or Therapeutic Category or Drug	Rationale	Recommendation	Quality/ Strength
Nitrofurantoin	Potential for pulmonary toxicity, hepatotoxicity, and peripheral neuropathy, especially with long-term use; safer alternatives available	**Avoid** for long-term suppression e.g. chronic UTIs; avoid in pts with low GFR	Low/Strong

The anti-infective agent nitrofurantoin (Macrodantin / Macrobid®) is the only anti-infective agent on the Beers list (Table 7.7). It has long been known that Macrobid® increases the potential for pulmonary toxicity (diffuse interstitial pneumonitis or pulmonary fibrosis, or both) and this increases if the agent is used chronically. It is also known to cause hepatotoxicity and peripheral neuropathy when used chronically. There is also a lack of evidence in long-term suppression in chronic UTIs. In addition, it is best to avoid nitrofurantoin in patients with an *approximate* GFR < 50mL/min/1.73m^2 (CrCl <30 mL/min) since a strong concentration in the urine is required for the drug to work effectively.

At this point, it is important to note that we have been driven to believe that altered mental status (AMS) in the elderly is suggestive of a urinary tract infection; in reality it may not be. Nobel laureate Daniel Hahneman explained why "old habits" are hard to overcome. As human beings when we go through a decision-making process, we draw off of two systems. System one is a **FAST** process and it's also an intuitive system; we use this system from immediately available information – such as the patient has an altered mental status – drawing an immediate conclusion of the anticipated problem. System two is a **SLOW** and deliberate process which uses questioning and further investigation.[59]

System one historically makes people feel comfortable and secure since those decisions are made based on what we interpret as facts. However, system one is only founded in past experience; it's like a reflex. Research has shown us this process correlates with predictable mistakes. System two, on the other hand, is founded in evidence. In a clinician's case, system two correlates with evidence-based medicine and is founded on reflection and logical thinking (Figure 7.1)

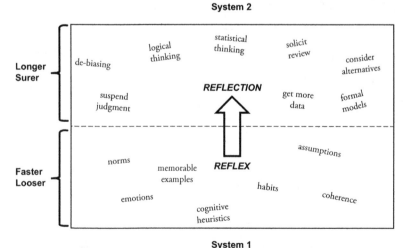

Figure 7.1: Systems of Human Decision Making

The first thought: if a patient has altered mental status, then they must have a urinary tract infection (UTI). Both families and medical personnel alike are drawn into the façade of this reflexive system. In fact, evidence-based medicine shows us infectious causes of delirium are the third most likely cause of that altered mental status, while medications and dehydration are much more common causes of that delirium.[60]

In 1991, McGeer and colleagues proposed an infection surveillance definition for long-term care facilities (LTCFs). Their intent was to provide standardized information for suspected infection using evidence-based medicine. In fact, these definitions became a standard of care and were adopted by infectious disease physicians, geriatricians, and infection control nurses with experience in LTCFs. These consensus definitions, also known as the McGeer criteria, were retested by Stone in 2012 to see if they still held true.[61] One of the reasons it was done however, was to debunk the myth that altered mental status is caused by a UTI. (Figure 7.2).

A diagnosis of a UTI in non-catheterized patients, as is noted from the McGeer Criteria, should satisfy both criteria in order to warrant treatment. Criterion 1 focuses only on the signs and symptoms. Criterion 2 focuses on the microbiology report from the culture and sensitivity.

In Criterion 1, a patient should present with acute dysuria or pain, swelling or tenderness of the testes, epididymis or prostate. If this is absent, the patient can present with fever or leukocytosis plus any one of the following:

- Acute CVA pain or tenderness
- Suprapubic pain
- Gross hematuria
- New or marked increase in incontinence
- New or marked increase in urgency
- New or marked increase in frequency

In the absence of fever or leukocytosis, any two of the bulleted items should be present.

If Criterion 1 is met, using what was discussed above, then send a urine sample out for a culture and sensitivity. Otherwise, this author recommends considering if medications or dehydration contributed to the changes in mental status, since these are the two most likely and more common causes.

Diagnosis of UTIs in Nursing Home Residents

Noncatheterized patients must satisfy Criteria 1 *and* 2 to meet UTI criteria:

CRITERIA #1

At least 1 of the following signs/ symptoms:

   A. Acute dysuria or pain, swelling or tenderness of testes, epididymis or prostate
   B. Fever or leukocytosis + at least one of these localizing criteria:
        i. Acute CVA Pain or Tenderness
        ii. Suprapubic Pain
        iii. Gross Hematuria
        iv. New or marked increase in incontinence
        v. New or marked increase in urgency
        vi. New or marked increase in frequency
   C. If no fever or leukocytosis, 2 or more from items ii – vi, above, are documented

IF Criteria #1, above, is met and documented, check a UA

CRITERIA #2

One of the following two microbiologic subcriteria:

   A.   >100,000 cfu/ml of no more than 2 species of microorganisms in a voided urine sample
   B.   >100,000 cfu/ml of any number of organisms in a specimen collected via catheter

If they meet both criteria, start an appropriate antibiotic

USEFUL INFORMATION ABOUT UTIs:

- Bacteria in the urine without meeting these criteria is usually **asymptomatic bacteriuria** and should **NOT** be treated
- Behavior change' or 'acting different' is not part of either criteria
- Increasing fluids is almost always a good idea, clearing the bladder of stagnant, microorganism-rich urine
- Overuse of antibiotics leads to resistant organisms, unnecessary and potentially dangerous side-effects, added cost, risks adverse drug events, and increasing prevalence of C-Dift

Monitor and assess patient's hydration status, to ensure they are consuming *plenty* of extra fluids

Figure 7.2: The McGeer Criteria

This author's hope is that EVERYONE will print Figure 7.2 and make it available to anyone who will accept it. Permission is granted to use, print and distribute Figure 7.2 without notification to the publisher or the author.

It shouldn't be surprising that cardiovascular agents make up the bulk of medications on the Beers criteria since they represent the most widely prescribed class of medications.

CARDIOVASCULAR MEDICATIONS

Table 7.8: Cardiovascular Agents

Organ System or Therapeutic Category or Drug	Rationale	Recommendation	Quality/Strength
Peripheral alpha-1 blockers			
Doxazosin Prazosin Terazosin	High risk of orthostatic hypotension; not recommended as routine treatment for HTN; alternative agents have superior risk/benefit profile.	**Avoid** use as an antihypertensive	Moderate/ Strong
Alpha agonists, central			
Clonidine Guanabenz Guanfacine Methyldopa Reserpine (>.1mg/d)	High risk of adverse CNS effects; may cause bradycardia and orthostatic hypotension; not recommended as routine treatment for hypertension.	**Avoid** clonidine as a first-line antihypertensive. Avoid others as listed.	Low/ Strong
Antiarrhythmic drugs			
Disopyramide	Potent negative inotrope and may induce heart failure in older adults; strongly anticholinergic; other antiarrhythmic drugs preferred.	**Avoid**	Low/ Strong
Dronedarone	Worse outcomes have been reported in patients taking dronedarone who have permanent atrial fibrillation or severe or recently decompensated heart failure.	**Avoid**	High/ Strong

Organ System or Therapeutic Category or Drug	Rationale	Recommendation	Quality/ Strength
Antiarrhythmic drugs			
Digoxin	Use in atrial fibrillation: should not be used as a first-line agent in atrial fibrillation, because more-effective alternatives exist and it may be associated with increased mortality.	**Avoid** as first-line therapy for atrial fibrillation.	Afib: Moderate/ Strong
	Use in heart failure: questionable effects on risk of hospitalization and may be associated with increased mortality in older adults with heart failure; in heart failure, higher dosages not associated with additional benefit and may increase risk of toxicity.	**Avoid** as first-line therapy for heart failure.	Heart Failure: Low/ Strong
	Decreased renal clearance of digoxin may lead to increased risk of toxic effects; further dose reduction may be necessary in patients with stage 4 or 5 CKD.	If used for atrial filbrillation or heart failure, **avoid** dosages >0.125mg/d.	Dosing: Moderate/ Strong
Nifedipine, immediate release	Potential for hypotension; risk of precipitating myocardial ischemia.	**Avoid**	High/ Strong

Organ System or Therapeutic Category or Drug	Rationale	Recommendation	Quality/ Strength
Antiarrhythmic drugs			
Amiodarone	Amiodarone is effective for maintaining sinus rhythm but has greater toxicities than other antiarrhythmics used in atrial fibrillation (including thyroid disease, pulmonary disorders, and QT-interval prolongation); it may be a reasonable first-line therapy in patients with concomitant heart failure or substantial left ventricular hypertrophy if rhythm control is preferred over rate control.	**Avoid** amiodarone as first-line therapy for atrial fibrillation unless patient has heart failure or substantial left ventricular hypertrophy.	High/ Strong

All of the alpha$_1$-blockers risk orthostatic hypotension and must be used in caution with any older adult. They do this because not only do they relax certain muscles (such as in the prostate) but they keep the small peripheral blood vessels open. Blocking the ability of those small peripheral blood vessels to constrict, in effect, causes the vessels to permanently remain open and relaxed, even when a person needs an increase in their blood pressures such as when they stand up.

Since alternative anti-hypertensive agents have superior risk/benefit profiles, the benefit should outweigh the risk if the medical provider decides to use these alpha$_1$-blockers. Incidentally, make note that in the Beers criteria, they are referencing alpha$_1$-blockers as they relate to blood pressure management and not for enlargement of the prostate. Needless to say, if they are used for hyperplasia of the prostate, the clinician should always consider what it may do to the patient's blood pressure. The quality of evidence to support this recommendation is moderate and the strength of the recommendation is strong.

In addition, many of the central acting alpha-agonists, clonidine (Catapress®) probably being one of the most common (Table 7.8), also risk severe orthostatic hypotension; as such these types of anti-hypertensives are implicated in a lot of falls. Additionally, in geriatric adults, they have also been implicated in adverse CNS effects, such as delirium, and cardiac effects such as bradycardia. The strength of the recommendation is strong; the quality of evidence has been shown to be low.

The antiarrhythmic agents pose a significant risk to patients. Those drug classes already have a high incidence of cardiac issues. Disopyramide (Norpace®), as a potent negative inotrope, has been shown to induce heart failure in older adults. It is also strongly anticholinergic. Consequently, other antiarrhythmic medications are preferred. Dronedarone (Multaq®) is another medication whose outcomes as an antiarrhythmic have been deemed inappropriate in the geriatric population. Both of these agents carry with them a strong recommendation.

The DIG (Digitalis Investigation Group) trial was a large study done in the 1980s. The goal of the study was to evaluate whether digoxin had a beneficial, harmful or no effect on total mortality in patients with clinical heart failure. Initially, the trial showed that adding digoxin had no effect on mortality and decreased hospitalizations related to heart failure and improved symptoms in patients treated for heart failure. However, in approximately 2006, a reanalysis was done on these data and it was shown that an increase in mortality occurred.[62] Since that time digoxin has appropriately fallen out of favor and higher dosages have not been shown to be associated with additional benefit and may increase risk of toxicity. The quality of evidence in heart failure is low, the recommendation from the panel is strong.

Additionally, digoxin should be avoided as first-line therapy in atrial fibrillation. Given the suggested risk of increased mortality, alternatives should be considered first. Even so, if digoxin is desired or needed, it should not be used in doses greater than 0.125mg (125mcg) because it has been associated with no additional benefit in either heart failure or atrial fibrillation.

Digoxin also risks toxicity, especially considering the risk of toxic effects and slow renal clearance in adults who already bring impaired renal clearance to the table. Dose reductions beyond 0.125mg (125mcg) may be needed in Stage IV or V chronic kidney disease (CKD).

Nifedipine (immediate release) has long been known to increase the risk of hypotension; it has also been known to precipitate myocardial ischemia.[63]

Both of those risks are now part of the package insert for nifedipine (Adalat® and Procardia®) and it is recommended to avoid this agent for treatment of immediate hypertension. It's important to note that this recommendation does not apply to the long-acting nifedipine.

Albeit, it is true that amiodarone has been shown to be an effective antiarrhythmic medication for the maintenance of sinus rhythm, but its use is limited by significant non-cardiovascular toxicities such as thyroid disease, pulmonary disorders and QT-interval prolongation. In addition, the half-life ranges between 40-60 days which poses additional risk to older adults. Randomized trials comparing rate control versus rhythm control strategies for the treatment of atrial fibrillation have demonstrated maintenance of sinus rhythm yields little to no added improvement in mortality.[64] More importantly, quality of life achieved little to no improvement over the rate control approach.[65] And unless the benefit outweighs the risk, amiodarone should be avoided unless a patient has heart failure or substantial left ventricular dysfunction. The quality of evidence that has been reviewed about amiodarone is high, and the strength of this recommendation is strong.

CENTRAL NERVOUS SYSTEM

Table 7.9: Agents Affecting the Central Nervous System

Organ System or Therapeutic Category or Drug	Rationale	Recommendation	Quality/ Strength
Antidepressants, alone or in combination			
• Amitriptyline • Amoxapine • Clomipramine • Desipramine • Doxepin > 6mg/d • Imipramine • Nortriptyline • Paroxetine • Protriptyline • Trimipramine	Highly anticholinergic, sedating, and cause orthostatic hypotension; safety profile of doxepin (≤6mg/d) is comparable with placebo.	**Avoid**	High/ Strong

Organ System or Therapeutic Category or Drug	Rationale	Recommendation	Quality/ Strength
Antipyschotics			
Antipsychotics, first (conventional) and second (atypical) generation	Increased risk of cerebrovascular accident (stroke) and greater rate of cognitive decline and mortality in persons with dementia. Avoid antipsychotics for behavioral problems of dementia or delirium unless nonpharmacological options (e.g., behavioral interventions) have failed or are not possible and the older adult is threatening substantial harm to self or others.	**Avoid**, except for schizophrenia, bipolar disorder, or short-term use as antiemetic during chemotherapy.	Moderate/ Strong
Barbiturates			
• Amobarbital • Butabarbital • Butalbital • Mephobarbital • Pentobarbital • Phenobarbital • Secobarbital	High rate of physical dependence; tolerance to sleep benefits; risk of overdose at low dosages.	**Avoid**	High/ Strong
Benzodiazepines (short/int'd acting)			
• Alprazolam • Estazolam • Lorazepam • Oxazepam • Temazepam • Triazolam	Older adults have increased sensitivity to BZDs and slower metabolism of long-acting agents. In general, all BZDs increase risk of cognitive impairment, delirium, falls, fractures, and motor vehicle accidents in older adults.	**Avoid**	Moderate/ Strong

Organ System or Therapeutic Category or Drug	Rationale	Recommendation	Quality/ Strength
Benzodiazepines (long-acting)			
• Clorazepate • Chlordiazepoxide (alone or in combination with amitriptyline or clidinium) • Clonazepam • Diazepam • Flurazepam • Quazepam	May be appropriate for seizure disorders, rapid eye movement sleep disorders, benzodiazepine withdrawal, ethanol withdrawal, severe generalized anxiety disorder, periprocedural anesthesia.	**Avoid**	Moderate/ Strong
Non-benzodiazepine, benzodiazepine receptor agonist hypnotics			
• Eszopiclone • Zolpidem • Zaleplon	High rate of physical dependence; very sedating. BZD-receptor agonists have adverse events similar to those of BZDs in older adults (delirium, falls, fractures); increased emergency department visits and hospitalizations; motor vehicle crashes; minimal improvement in sleep latency and duration.	**Avoid**	Moderate/ Strong
• Ergoloid mesylates (dehydrogenated ergot alkaloids) • Isoxsuprine	Lack of efficacy.	**Avoid**	High/ Strong

Delirium as a result of medications – especially those listed in Table 7.9 – is the most common culprit implicated in delirium in the elderly.[66] Clinical experience has clearly shown that delirium in older adults can initiate, or otherwise be a key component in, a cascade of events that lead to a downward spiral of permanent functional decline, loss of independence, institutionalization, and death. Delirium affects an estimated 14–56% of all hospitalized elderly patients.[67] The Beers criteria panel clearly understood the implications of agents that affect mental state. The medications listed in Table 7.9 should be evaluated carefully to determine if they are indeed appropriate for geriatric adults.

Tertiary tricyclic antidepressants (TCAs) have long been used in the setting of sleep disorders and depression. The rationale for their placement on the Beers criteria is that they are highly anticholinergic and are known to cause orthostatic hypotension and pose significant anticholinergic risks (Table 7.3) to older adults.[68] There are much safer and frankly, better alternatives to these agents. In general, avoid these agents, but should patients be on them, strong considerations should be made to both reduce (abrupt discontinuance should be avoided) and discontinue these agents. The quality of evidence for this recommendation is high and has been demonstrated over and over. The strength of the evidence to support it, strong.

Both first and second generation antipsychotic agents have long been known to pose significant risks to older adults. They do provide off-label benefit in the presence of dementia with behaviors in some circumstances but all are known to increase the risk of stroke and mortality in patients who are older and demented.[69] Additionally, they risk hyperglycemia and diabetes, hyperlipidemia, and falls.

The significance of mortality secondary to anti-psychotics in the literature from years past suggested that for every 100 patients who used either a typical or atypical antipsychotics, there was one medication-related death. Most recent literature showed this number is much more common. In 2003, the FDA issued a "black-box" warning on risperidone based on a multinational study that opened our eyes to the risk of these drugs and their association with death.[70]

Then, in 2005, Schneider et al. did a meta-analysis of 15 RCTs further expounding on that risk and demonstrating the number-needed-to-harm (NNH) – which indicates how many patients on average need to be exposed to a risk factor over a specific period to cause harm in one patient who would not otherwise have been harmed – was approximately 1 patient in every 100 patients. At the time of that study, however, evidence was unavailable regarding individual antipsychotics (risperidone, olanzapine, etc.), nor did it account for relationships or differences among dementia types.

To address this concern, the VA conducted a retrospective case-control study on patients from 1998 through 2009. Participants included nearly 91,000 patients, all were 65 years or older and 20% of those patients were over 85. All had a diagnosis of dementia. Final analysis was conducted in August 2014. Besides age, inclusion criteria for the study included being demented and a BRAND new prescription for a single antipsychotic (haloperidol, olanzapine, quetiapine, and risperidone), valproic acid and its derivatives, or an antidepressant. Forty-six thousand patients were noted to take one of those drugs, and 44,000 patients did not take any of these drugs. Additionally, the two groups were matched for age, sex, years with dementia, presence of delirium, as well as other clinical and demographic characteristics. Then they looked at absolute change in mortality risk, or, the NNH one patient over 180 days of follow-up. Secondary analysis was also done and compared a dose-adjusted absolute change in mortality risk for each of the four antipsychotics if the group was using them. The results were alarming!

The retrospective study showed that over 180 days of treatment, haloperidol (Haldol®) caused one death in every 26 patients, risperidone (Risperdal®) caused one death in every 27 patients, olanzapine (Zyprexa®) caused one death every 40 patients, and quetiapine (Seroquel®) caused one death in every 50 patients that it was used for.[71] This is representative of a two-to-four fold increase over the original study by Schnieder. Additionally, it appeared that valproate and its derivatives did not increase mortality. Moreover, it demonstrated that the risk of death is dose-related, suggesting that higher doses may be associated with additional mortality.

Nevertheless, it's important to note that certain patients do get benefits from these medications, though it is strongly encouraged that dose reductions be considered. This is especially true for patients in facilities that are known for managing behaviors adequately and may be able to use redirection as a non-pharmacological treatment approach.

It should be quite clear why barbiturates are listed on the Beers criteria. All barbiturates, but particularly those listed, have a high rate of physical dependence and tolerance. More importantly, there is a risk of overdose, even at low dosages. They should be avoided in geriatric adults.

All of the short-, intermediate-, and long-acting benzodiazepines (BZDs) risk cognitive impairment, delirium and falls in the older patient. The most important risk is fractures that can occur when these medications are prescribed.[72] There is no doubt these medications play a very important BENEFICIAL role when patients are at risk for harming themselves, or others, and require control of that behavior. However, these medications should be used prudently and, most importantly, over as short a course as possible! It should be noted though, these medications may be appropriate and necessary in the setting of seizure disorders, benzodiazepine withdrawal, ethanol withdrawal, periprocedural anesthesia and end-of-life. They can also be used routinely for severe generalized anxiety disorder (GAD) should other psychological treatments (pharmacological and non-pharmacological) fail. As an example, other safer agents (such as SSRIs and SNRIs) should be considered since long-term management over time with benzodiazepines can lead to tolerance, dependence and dementia.

Meprobamate (marketed under the trade name Miltown®) was a best-selling anxiolytic drug before the advent of benzodiazepines. It has well been known to have a high degree of physical dependence and is very sedating. It is recommended to avoid its use in geriatric adults.[73]

The non-benzodiazepine hypnotics include the sleeping medications eszopiclone (Lunesta®), zolpidem (Ambien®) and zeleplon (Sonata®). They have long been known to cause serious side-effects in the elderly including delirium, falls and fractures.[74] Also, they produce only minimal improvement in sleep latency and duration.[75] Chronic use of these medications can lead to dependency. As a general rule, when medications increase delirium, falls and fractures, they are best avoided in geriatrics.

Ergoloid mesylates, which is also an ergot alkaloid, became famous for their ability to increase cerebral metabolism and blood flow. Their role was thought to improve outcomes in dementia, particularly vascular dementia or ischemic strokes. Controlled studies in patients with Alzheimer's disease found there was no advantage to the use of ergoloid mesylates compared to placebo; some studies suggest they may lower scores on some cognitive and behavioral rating scales. Further study is needed to determine the risk-benefit profile of ergoloid mesylates in the treatment of dementia, but no benefit has been demonstrated to date in geriatric adults. Examples of trade names for this drug include Hydergine®, Hydergina®, Gerimal®, Niloric®, Redizork®, Alkergot®, Cicanol®, and Redergin®.

ENDOCRINE SYSTEM

Table 7.10: The Endocrine System

Organ System or Therapeutic Category or Drug	Rationale	Recommendation	Quality/ Strength
Androgens			
Methyltestosterone Testosterone	Potential for cardiac problem and contraindicated in men with prostate CA.	**Avoid** unless indicated for confirmed hypogonadism with symptoms.	Moderate/ Weak

Organ System or Therapeutic Category or Drug	Rationale	Recommendation	Quality/ Strength
Androgens			
Desiccated thyroid	Concerns about cardiac effects; safer alternatives available.	**Avoid**	Low/Strong
Estrogens with or without progestins	Evidence of carcinogenic potential (breast and endometrium); lack of cardioprotective effect and cognitive protection in older women. Evidence indicates that vaginal estrogens for the treatment of vaginal dryness are safe and effective; women with a history of breast cancer who do not respond to non-hormonal therapies are advised to discuss the risk and benefits of low-dose vaginal estrogen (dosages of estradiol <25 μg twice weekly) with their healthcare provider.	**Avoid** oral and topical patch. Vaginal cream or tablets: acceptable to use low-dose intravaginal estrogen for management of dyspareunia, lower urinary tract infections, and other vaginal symptoms.	Oral and patch: High/ Strong Vaginal Cream or Tablets: Moderate / Weak

Organ System or Therapeutic Category or Drug	Rationale	Recommendation	Quality/ Strength
Androgens			
Growth hormone	Impact on body composition is small and associated with edema, arthralgia, carpal tunnel syndrome, gynecomastia, impaired fasting glucose.	**Avoid** except as hormone replacement after pituitary gland removal.	High/Strong
Insulin, sliding scale	Higher risk of hypoglycemia without improvement in hyperglycemia management **regardless of care setting**; refers to sole use of short- or rapid-acting insulins to manage or avoid hyperglycemia in absence of basal or long-acting insulin; does not apply to titration of basal insulin or use of additional short- or rapid-acting insulin in conjunction with scheduled insulin (i.e., correction insulin).	**Avoid**	Moderate/ Strong

Organ System or Therapeutic Category or Drug	Rationale	Recommendation	Quality/ Strength
Androgens			
Megestrol	Minimal effect on weight; increases risk of thrombotic events and possibly death in older adults.	**Avoid**	Moderate/ Strong
Sulfonylureas, long-duration			
Chlorpropamide	Prolonged half-life causing prolonged hypoglycemia; causes SIADH.	**Avoid**	High/Strong
Glyburide	Greater risk of prolonged hypoglycemia in older adults.	**Avoid**	High/Strong

Androgens were a new category in Beers 2012 but certainly they are newsworthy items given the amount of controversy they have sparked in the last 5 years or so. Methyltestosterone and testosterone are the two that are listed. The rationale for their placement on the Beers criteria is their potential for cardiac problems and their contraindication in men with prostate cancer (a risk that increases with age). They also risk blood clots as is noted in the package insert.

Desiccated thyroid refers to porcine (or mixed beef and pork) thyroid for therapeutic use. It is commonly known as "Armour thyroid." Geriatricians have long known there are safer alternatives available due to concerns about cardiac effects of desiccated thyroid. It should be pointed out the quality of evidence is low, but the strength of the recommendation is strong for desiccated thyroid.

Since the HERS[76] trial (the Heart Estrogen/Progestin Replacement Study) and the WHI[77] (Women's Health Initiative), estrogens with or without progestins have been known to be risky in older adults due to the lack of cardioprotective effects they were once touted to have. Additionally, the cardiogenic potential poses a significant risk. This applies to both the oral forms and patch forms of estrogen. The topical vaginal creams, however, pose less risk to patients, especially for the management of dyspareunia and lower urinary tract symptoms (LUTS) and can be used without the same risk.

Growth hormones are associated with risks like edema, generalized arthralgia, carpal tunnel syndrome, gynecomastia and impaired fasting glucose levels. The quality of the evidence is high and the strength of the recommendation is strong. It is recommended to be avoided unless a patient has had a pituitary gland removal.

Insulin sliding scales (SSI), in the setting of long-term care especially, poses significant risks of hypoglycemia which can be potentially lethal for older adults. Studies have shown us that this is relevant **no matter what care setting** the patient is in – hospital, subacute care, long-term care, etc.[78] Studies have also given us a clearer picture of the real risk of mortality associated with tight HgA$_1$c control. For those with tighter control, a HgA$_1$c of less than 6.5%, death rates are approximately 20% higher in the geriatric population.[79] In fact, 5 long-term studies – ADOPT[80], DREAM[81], RECORD[82], ACCORD[83], VADT[84] – suggest no improvement in total mortality with tighter overall sugar control. Given the risk of death associated with tight HgA$_1$c control, individualized care plans are needed when older adults are diabetic, and frailty must be taken into consideration. This recommendation is strong due to the risk, and the quality of the evidence is moderate. As time goes by, the evidence has been mounting against tight diabetic control in our seniors.

Additional anti-glycemic agents that should be avoided include the long-acting sulfonylureas since they also increase the risk of hypoglycemia.[85] Two long-acting secretagogues are on the Beers Criteria. Chlorpropamide (Diabinese®) and glyburide (DiaBeta®; Micronase®) are known to have long half-lives—36 hours and 10 hours respectively—compared to glipizide (Glucotrol®) which has a half-life of approximately 2.5 hours. Additionally, chlorpropamide is known to cause the syndrome of inappropriate antidiuretic hormone (SIADH) secretion. As a consequence of the significant risks associated with hypoglycemia in the elderly, short-acting agents should be chosen if secretagogues are used.

SIADH is a disorder of impaired water excretion. Should water intake exceed urine output, the ensuing water retention leads to the development of hyponatremia. In older adults, hyponatremia is common but usually benign. Serum sodium levels of greater than or equal to 130mEq/L and less than 135mEq/L rarely pose a concern, but below this level older adults may complain of headache, nausea, vomiting, and confusion may ensue. As levels drop below 125mEq/L, more severe signs occur such as lethargy, fatigue, loss of appetite, irritability, muscle weakness, and spasms or cramps. Even lower numbers can lead to seizures, decreased consciousness, coma or even death.

GASTROINTESTINAL SYSTEM

Table 7.11: The Gastrointestinal System

Organ System or Therapeutic Category or Drug	Rationale	Recommendation	Quality/ Strength
Metoclopramide	Can cause extrapyramidal effects (EPS) including tardive dyskinesia; risk may be greater in frail older adults.	**Avoid** unless for gastroparesis.	Moderate/ Strong
Mineral oil, given orally	Potential for aspiration and adverse effects; safer alternative available.	**Avoid**	Moderate/ Strong
Proton-pump inhibitors	Risk of *Clostridium difficile* infection and bone loss and fractures.	**Avoid** scheduled use for >8 weeks unless for high-risk patients (e.g., oral corticosteroids or chronic NSAID use), erosive esophagitis, Barrett's esophagitis, pathological hypersecretory condition, or demonstrated need for maintenance treatment (e.g., due to failure of drug discontinuation trial or H_2 blockers)	High/Strong

Three medications made the Beers criteria for the GI system in 2015. They include metoclopramide (Reglan®), oral mineral oils, and proton-pump inhibitors (Aciphex®, Dexilant®, Kapidex®, Nexium®, Prilosec®, Protonix®, Zegerid®).

Metoclopramide (Reglan®), an agent known to cause extrapyramidal symptoms (EPS) and tardive dyskinesia (TD)[86], should generally be avoided as a consequence of this risk. Extrapyramidal symptoms (EPS) are drug-induced movement disorders whose symptoms include dystonia (continuous spasms and muscle contractions), akathisia (motor restlessness), and parkinsonism (characteristic symptoms such as rigidity, bradykinesia, and tremor). Tardive dyskinesia is associated with involuntary, repetitive body movements of the face, torso and limbs. Both EPS and TD can persist in the presence of metoclopramide but, more importantly, both can be permanent. Since metoclopramide was originally prescribed for gastroesophageal reflux (GERD), nausea, or vomiting, and newer medications have been developed since, the risk of EPS is high enough that it should be avoided if possible. The one consideration where Reglan may be an option is gastroparesis. However, even in this case, Reglan should be discontinued as soon as feasible, given the high rates of side effects.

Historically, patients were prescribed mineral oils for constipation. It is well-known as a lubricant laxative. It works by keeping water in the stool and intestines. However, oral mineral oils have been known to potentiate aspiration pneumonia and certainly, for constipation, safer alternative are available.[87]

Proton-pump inhibitors (PPIs) have been newly added to the 2015 Beers criteria though they have been on STOPP/START for some time (see Chapter 9). Proton-pump inhibitors are often prescribed to minimize the risk of GI hemorrhage which can occur in times of stress such as admission into the hospital. This then turns into a lasting prescription after discharge. The maximum recommended treatment duration for many of these indications is 8 weeks[88] and shorter if the intent for use was only prophylaxis. In order to prevent prolonged inappropriate use, evaluation of symptom resolution and need for continued therapy should be performed. But the risks of overuse are alarming.

In 2012, a meta-analysis of 42 observational studies that included 313,000 patients found that PPI use was significantly associated with an increased risk of both incident and recurrent C. difficile (Cdiff) infections.[89] And, the incidence of Cdiff increases the risk of death markedly. Approximately 29,000 patients died in 2011 within 30 days of the initial diagnosis of C. difficile. More than 80 percent of those were deaths were amongst those aged 65 years or older.[90]

In addition, PPIs are also strongly associated with an increased risk of community-acquired pneumonia[91], malabsorption of key minerals in the body, namely calcium and magnesium[92], and patients who take PPIs for extended periods of time (>1 year) are more likely to experience a fracture.[93]

The quality of the evidence for the recommendations in the Beers criteria is high, and the strength of the recommendation is strong, such that clinicians should avoid scheduled PPIs for >8 weeks unless that patient is considered high risk. Examples of patients who may require longer use PPIs, include those taking oral corticosteroids or chronic NSAIDs. It may also include those with erosive esophagitis, Barrett's esophagitis, pathological hypersecretory conditions, or those who demonstrate the need for maintenance treatment such as failure of a PPI discontinuation trial or failure of a H_2 blocker.

Most recently, a new study has identified a possible link between proton pump inhibitors (PPIs) and dementia in older adults.[94] In a prospective cohort study of >73,000 geriatric adults (≥75 years) who were free of dementia at baseline but regularly used PPIs was associated with a 1.4-fold increase in the risk of incident dementia, independent of age, gender, depression, stroke, heart disease, and polypharmacy. Since this was only one study, and it was prospective rather than double-blinded, more studies are needed to confirm or refute this association.

ANALGESICS

Table 7.12: Analgesics

Organ System or Therapeutic Category or Drug	Rationale	Recommendation	Quality/ Strength
Meperidine	Not an effective oral analgesic in dosages commonly used; may have higher risk of neurotoxicity, including delirium, than other opioids; safer alternative available.	**Avoid** especially in individuals with CKD.	Moderate/ Strong

Organ System or Therapeutic Category or Drug	Rationale	Recommendation	Quality/ Strength
Non-COX-selective NSAIDs, oral			
• ASA > 325mg/d • Diclofenac • Diflunisal • Etodolac • Fenoprofen • Ibuprofen • Ketoprofen • Meclofenamate • Mefenamic acid • Meloxicam • Nabumetone • Naproxen • Oxaprozin • Piroxicam • Sulindac • Tolmetin	Increases risk of GI bleeding and PUD in high-risk groups, including those aged > 75 or taking orals or parenteral corticosteroids, anticoagulants, or antiplatelet agents. Use of PPI or misoprostol reduces but doesn't eliminate risk. Upper GI ulcers, gross bleeding or perforation by NSAIDs occur in approximately 1% of patients treated for 3-6 months and in approximately 2-4% of patients for 1 year. These trends continue with longer duration of use.	**Avoid** chronic use unless other alternatives are not effective and patient can take GI protective agent (PPI or misoprostol).	Moderate/ Strong

Organ System or Therapeutic Category or Drug	Rationale	Recommendation	Quality/ Strength
Indomethacin, Ketorolac, including parenteral	Indomethacin is more likely than other NSAIDs to have adverse CNS effects. Of all the NSAIDs, indomethacin has the most adverse effects. Increased risk of gastrointestinal bleeding, peptic ulcer disease, and acute kidney injury in older adults. Ketorolac increases the risk of GI hemorrhage and PUD in high-risk groups.	**Avoid**	Moderate/ Strong
Pentazocine	Opioid analgesic that causes CNS adverse effects, including confusion and hallucinations, more commonly than other narcotic drugs; is also a mixed agonist and antagonist; safer alternatives available.	**Avoid**	Low/ Strong

Organ System or Therapeutic Category or Drug	Rationale	Recommendation	Quality/ Strength
Skeletal Muscle Relaxant			
• Carisoprodol • Chlorzoxazone • Cyclobenzaprine • Metaxaolone • Methocarbamol • Orphenadrine	Most muscle relaxants are poorly tolerated by older adults because of the anticholinergic adverse effects, sedation, risk of fracture; effectiveness at dosages tolerated by older adults is questionable.	**Avoid**	Moderate/ Strong

The MAJORITY of analgesics that pose a significant risk to older adults are NSAIDs. Non-steroidal anti-inflammatory drugs (including aspirin in doses greater than 325mg daily) markedly increase the risk of GI hemorrhage and peptic-ulcer disease (PUD). The highest risk groups are patients older than 75 years of age or those who use concomitant corticosteroids, anticoagulants or anti-platelet agents.

Though proton-pump inhibitors (PPIs) or misoprostol reduce the risk of GI hemorrhage, they do not eliminate the risk. According to the Beers criteria, upper GI ulcers, gross bleeding or perforation by NSAIDs occur in approximately 1% of patients treated for 3-6 months and 2-4% of patients treated for 1 year. These trends continue the longer the duration of NSAID use.

The recommendation is to avoid NSAIDs, even acutely, unless other alternatives are not effective. If a patient insists on, or must, use NSAID therapy, then PPIs or misoprostol need to be initiated at the same time to minimize the risk of GI hemorrhage.

The risk of heart attack and stroke (the leading causes of death amongst the elderly) with NSAIDs, was first described in 2005 in the boxed warning and Warnings and Precautions sections of the prescription drug label for NSAIDs. Since then, a large combined analysis of clinical trials, observational studies and other scientific publications has been done. Initially, those estimates suggested that 6-12 months of NSAID use increased risk, we now know the estimates of increased risk range from 10 percent to 50 percent or more, depending on the drugs and the doses studied, and may occur as early as the first weeks of treatment and also increase with duration of use.[95]

The other two analgesic agents on the Beers criteria include indomethacin (Indocin®) and ketorolac (Toradol®). Both of these agents increase the risk of GI hemorrhage and PUD. Additionally, indomethacin is associated with other adverse events which are primarily psychiatric in nature: agitation, anxiety, pseudo-dementia, psychosis, depression and hallucinations.[96]

Meperidine (Demerol®) has long been known to be potentially dangerous in the elderly. It has not been shown to be as effective an agent for pain management as other comparable analgesics. More importantly it may cause neurotoxicity, which can lead to seizures.

Pentazocine (Talwin®) is an opioid analgesic that causes adverse CNS effects including hallucinations and other psychomimetic effects higher than those found with comparable analgesic agents. Since it's a mixed agonist and antagonist, efficacy varies. Quite simply, there are safer alternatives available. The recommendation is to avoid this agent; however, the quality of evidence is low since this agent is such an old analgesic, but the recommendation it comes with is strong.

The skeletal muscle relaxants are also agents that are commonly poorly tolerated by older adults because of their anticholinergic side-effects. However, the agents listed in the Beers criteria (Soma®, Parafon®, Flexeril® as examples) can also increase sedation and have been associated with an increased risk of fractures.[97] It is best to avoid these agents given the strong recommendation. There are three skeletal muscle relaxants that are not on the Beers criteria. Tizanidine (Zanaflex®), baclofen (Lioresal®), dantrolene (Dantrium®) are three muscle relaxants that may be considered in the elderly. They still have side effects, but these effects are not nearly as severe as those noted in Table 7.12.

GENITOURINARY SYSTEM

Table 7.13: Genitourinary System

Organ System or Therapeutic Category or Drug	Rationale	Recommendation	Quality/ Strength
Desmopressin	High risk of hyponatremia; safer alternative treatments.	**Avoid** for treatment of nocturia or nocturnal polyuria.	Moderate/ Strong

Desmopressin is a hormone that works by limiting the amount of water that is eliminated in the urine. Normally, desmopressin is used in diabetes insipidus but it can also be used to control excessive thirst or after a head injury or certain types of surgery. In children, desmopressin is used to control bed-wetting but it should not be used for this purpose in older adults due to the high risk of hyponatremia (see risk of hyponatremia described under the endocrine system above).

One of the new additions in the 2015 criteria is a list of 13 select drug-drug interactions (excluding anti-infective medication related interactions).[98] Although this list is not meant to diminish what was extensively detailed in Chapters 5 and 6, these interactions have specific evidence of causing serious harm in older adults if overlooked.

Table 7.14: Clinically Important Non-Anti-Infective Drug-Drug Interactions

Drug A	Drug B	Risk Rationale	Recommendation
ACEIs	Amiloride or triamterene	Increased risk of hyperkalemia	**Avoid** routine use
Anticholinergics	**ALL** Anticholinergics	Increased risk of cognitive decline	**Avoid** routine use or minimize number
Antidepressant	≥2 other CNS-active drugs	Increased risk of falls	**Avoid** 3 or more CNS-active drugs; minimize use
Antipsychotics		Increased risk of falls	
Hypnotics		Increased risk of falls and fractures	
Opioid analgesics		Increased risk of falls	
Corticosteroids (oral or parenteral)	NSAIDs	Increased risk of GI bleeding / peptic ulcer disease (PUD)	**Avoid**; if not possible, provide GI protection
Lithium	ACE inhibitors and/or loop diuretics	Increased risk of lithium toxicity	**Avoid**; if using monitor lithium concentration

Drug A	Drug B	Risk Rationale	Recommendation
Peripheral Alpha-1 blockers	Loop diuretics	Increased urinary incontinence in older women	**Avoid** in older women
Theophylline	Cimetidine	Increased risk of theophylline toxicity	**Avoid**
Warfarin	Amiodorone	Increased risk of bleeding	**Avoid** when possible; monitor closely if used together
	NSAIDs		

CHAPTER 8

Drug-Disease or Drug-Syndrome Interactions

As important as individual medications are to the Beers criteria, so too are drug-disease interactions or drug-syndrome interactions. The table that follows lists some of the most common in geriatric adults.

INAPPROPRIATE MEDICATIONS DUE TO DRUG-DISEASE OR DRUG-SYNDROME INTERACTIONS

Table 8.1: Inappropriate Medications Due to Drug-Disease or Drug-Syndrome Interactions

Disease or Syndrome	Drug(s)	Recommendation
Cardiovascular		
Heart Failure	• NSAIDs and COX-2 inhibitors • Non-dihydropyridine CCBs (diltiazem, verapamil) – avoid only for heart failure with reduced ejection fraction • TZDs (pioglitazone, rosiglitazone) • Cilostazol • Dronedarone (severe or recently decompensated heart failure)	Potential to increase fluid retention and exacerbate heart failure.

Disease or Syndrome	Drug(s)	Recommendation
Cardiovascular		

Syncope	• Acetylcholinesterase (ChI) inhibitors (donepezil, rivastigmine, galantamine)
	• Peripheral alpha$_1$-blockers
	  doxazosin
	  prazosin
	  terazosin
	• Tertiary TCAs
	• Chlorpromazine
	• Thioridazine
	• Olanzapine
		Increases the risk of orthostatic hypotension or bradycardia.

Central Nervous System		
Chronic seizures or epilepsy	• Bupropion • Chlorpromazine • Clozapine • Maprotiline • Olanzapine • Thioridazine • Thiothixene • Tramadol	Lower seizure threshold; may be acceptable in individuals with well-controlled seizures in whom alternative agents have not been effective.
Delirium	• Anticholinergics • Antipsychotics • Benzodiazepines • Chlorpromazine • Corticosteroids • H$_2$-receptor antagonists • Meperidine • Sedative hypnotics	Avoid in older adults with, or at high risk of, delirium because of the potential of inducing or worsening delirium. Avoid antipsychotics for behavioral problems of dementia or delirium unless nonpharmacological options (e.g., behavioral interventions) have failed or are not possible and the older adult is threatening substantial harm to self or others. Antipsychotics are associated with greater risk of stroke and mortality in persons with dementia.

Disease or Syndrome	Drug(s)	Recommendation
Central Nervous System		

Dementia or cognitive impairment	• Anticholinergics
	• Antipsychotics – chronic and as-needed use
	• Benzodiazepines (BZDs)
	• H$_2$-receptor antagonists
	• Hypnotics
	   eszopiclone (Lunesta®)
	   zolpidem (Ambien®)
	   zaleplon (Sonata®)
		Avoid because of adverse CNS effects.
		Avoid antipsychotics for behavioral problems of dementia or delirium unless nonpharmacological options (e.g., behavioral interventions) have failed or are not possible **and** the older adult is threatening substantial harm to self or others. Antipsychotics are associated with greater risk of cerebrovascular accident (stroke) and mortality in persons with dementia.

History of falls or fractures	• Anticonvulsants
	• Antipsychotics
	• Benzodiazepines (BZDs)
	• H$_2$-receptor antagonists
	• Hypnotics
	   eszopiclone (Lunesta®)
	   zolpidem (Ambien®)
	   zaleplon (Sonata®)
	• TCAs
	• SSRIs
	• Opioids
		May cause ataxia, impaired psychomotor function, syncope, falls; shorter-acting BZDs are not safer than long-acting ones. If one of the drugs must be used, consider reducing use of other CNS-active medications that increase risk of falls and fractures (e.g., anticonvulsants, benzodiazepine receptor agonists, other sedatives and hypnotics) and implement other strategies to reduce fall risk.
		Avoid unless safer alternatives are not available; avoid anticonvulsants except for seizure and mood disorders
		In the case of opioids, excludes pain management due to recent fractures or joint replacement.

Disease or Syndrome	Drug(s)	Recommendation
Central Nervous System		
Insomnia	• Oral decongestants pseudoephedrine phenylephrine • Stimulants amphetamine armodafinil methylphenidate modafinil • Theobromines theophylline caffeine	CNS stimulant effects
Parkinson's Disease	• All antipsychotics (except aripiprazole, quetiapine, clozapine) • Antiemetics metoclopramide prochlorperazine promethazine	Dopamine-receptor antagonist with potential to worsen parkinsonian symptoms Quetiapine, aripiprazole, and clozapine appear to be less likely to precipitate worsening of Parkinson's disease
Gastrointestinal		
History of gastric or duodenal ulcers	• Aspirin (>325mg/day) • Non-COX-2 selective NSAIDs	May exacerbate existing ulcers or cause new or additional ulcers Avoid unless other alternative ineffective. Start PPI or misoprostol if using
Kidney and Urinary Tract		
CKD stages IV or V	• NSAIDs (non-COX and COX-selective oral and parenteral)	May increase risk of acute kidney injury (AKI) and further decline of renal function
Urinary Incontinence (all types) in women	• Estrogen oral and transdermal (excludes intravaginal estrogen) • Peripheral alpha$_1$-blockers doxazosin prazosin terazosin	Aggravation of incontinence

Disease or Syndrome	Drug(s)	Recommendation
Kidney and Urinary Tract		
Lower urinary tract symptoms, benign prostatic hyperplasia	• Strongly anticholinergic drugs except antimuscarinic for urinary incontinence	May decrease urinary flow and cause urinary retention

In heart failure, it's important to avoid drugs that promote fluid retention which would thereby exacerbate heart failure. NSAIDs, including COX-2's, are included in the list. Diltiazem and verapamil are non-dihydropyridine calcium channel blockers (CCBs) which can be potentially dangerous medications especially in systolic heart failure; they can worsen congestive heart failure (CHF). Pioglitizone (Actos®) and rosiglitazone (Avandia®) are traditionally used in diabetes. They also promote fluid retention. Cilostazol (Pletal®) as well as dronedarone (Multaq®) are additional common examples of medications that can promote heart failure in geriatrics.

Syncope is precisely defined as a transient loss of consciousness and postural tone characterized by rapid onset and short duration. The layman's term for this is fainting. Beers 2015 looked at several classes of medications that may create a syncopal or syncopal-type episode. The acetylcholinesterase inhibitors (better known as the cognitive enhancers which include Aricept®, Exelon®, and Razadyne®) are a class of medications that can and do result in syncope. Given that people with dementia are at a risk of falls, it is important to recognize that if falls in an elderly demented adult occur, a provider should consider whether those medications are worth the risk. It should also be pointed out that these medications are not on the "Beers list," but on the list of agents that have the ability to *exacerbate* a disease or symptom. Additionally, the peripheral alpha$_1$-blockers doxazosin, prazosin and terazosin – usually used for prostatic hypertrophy – can cause syncope. As can nearly all of the tertiary TCAs. Phenothiazine antipsychotics are dopamine$_2$ (D$_2$) receptor antagonists therefore decrease the effect of dopamine in the brain. These classes of medications are better known as typical antipsychotics and are used to treat schizophrenia or psychosis. Chlorpromazine (Thorazine®) and thioridazine (Mellaril®) are common examples and are known to increase the risk of syncope and/or bradycardia. All second generation antipsychotics are known to cause syncope too. In geriatrics there are several medications affecting the CNS that lower a patient's seizure threshold. Common medications that are often overlooked as worsening a drug-syndrome interaction include buproprion (Wellbutrin®) and tramadol (Ultram®). Both of these medications lower the seizure threshold. It is best to avoid these medications in geriatrics if an underlying seizure disorder exists. Additionally, first-generation antipsychotics – clozapine (Clozaril®), thiordazine (Mellaril®), thiothixine (Navane®) – mono-amine oxidase inhibitors (MAOIs) which are one of the first anti-depressant classes ever created – maprotiline (Ludiomil®) – and second generation antipsychotics—olanzapine (Zyprexa®) and clozapine (Clozaril) – are also implicated in lowering the seizure threshold to increase this risk.

Delirium is another common side-effect of many medications. As has been discussed, anticholinergic agents are probably the worst offenders. But so too are first- and second-generation antipsychotics, tricyclic antidepressants, benzodiazepines, oral corticosteroids, H_2-antagonists (Zantac®, Pepcid®), meperidine (Demerol®) and sedative hypnotics. As was discussed earlier, delirium in the elderly can be lethal.

Additional CNS effects can worsen dementia and cognitive impairment. It is always appropriate to attempt non-pharmacological approaches to care for these patients since medications such as anticholinergics agents, benzodiazepines like lorazepam and alprazolam, H_2-antagonists, antipsychotics (chronic and as-needed use) and sedative hypnotics, can worsen memory. Furthermore, as has been stated earlier, antipsychotics have long been associated with an increased risk of stroke and mortality in older adults with dementia. They should only be used as a last resort (both long-term and short-term).

Falls and fractures are very serious side-effects of some medications. Those listed in Beers 2015 are duly noted for their adverse effects in causing falls (anticonvulsants, antipsychotics, benzodiazepines, non-benzodiazepine hypnotic agents (e.g., Ambien®, Lunesta®, and Sonata®), tricyclic antidepressants (e.g., Elavil®), newer-generation antidepressants (e.g., Prozac®, and Zoloft® and Effexor® and Cymbalta®), and opioids). As a general rule, when a medication carries risks of falls and fractures, every effort should be made to avoid or reduce their use. It should be noted that anticonvulsants do provide benefit for both seizures and mood disorders and there may be times when the risk does not outweigh the benefit in their use.

The prevalence of insomnia increases with age. A very common feature of insomnia in the elderly is the presence of anxiety and depression, so they must be ruled out. One study found that depression was as high as 69% in those with insomnia, and anxiety was as high as 61% in those with insomnia.[99] Common medications that contribute to insomnia include any oral decongestants, stimulants, and theobromines such as theophylline and caffeine. They should be avoided in the presence of insomnia.

Patients with Parkinson's disease should avoid medications that worsen their parkinsonian symptoms. Nearly all of the antipsychotics, except aripiprazole, quetiapine and clozapine, worsen these symptoms because they are dopamine-receptor antagonists. Additional agents that worsen these symptoms include metoclopramide, prochlorperazine, and promethazine.

When it comes to the gastrointestinal system, most all NSAIDS – except non-COX-2 selective NSAIDs – can exacerbate the risk of GI bleeding. Aspirin (ASA) also raises that risk and the risk is dose-related. Doses of ASA greater than 325mg/day should be avoided as is noted in the Beers criteria.

The final body system to discuss is the kidneys. There have been several discussions in the preceding chapters regarding the risks associated with many medications and the harm they can do to the kidney.

In Stage IV and V chronic kidney disease (CKD), non-COX NSAIDs should be avoided since they may risk inducing renal failure. Because of the large number of patients who take NSAIDs (estimates of more than 70 million prescriptions and 30 billion over-the-counter doses annually), this translates to upwards of 2.5 million patients experiencing a nephrotoxic event annually.[100] If these medications had to undergo the same scrutiny that newer drugs must undergo with the FDA, this author wonders if they would be allowed or not, given that risk.

CHAPTER 9

STOPP and START Criteria

STOPP (Screening Tool of Older Persons' Prescriptions) and START (Screening Tool to Alert to Right Treatment) were formulated to identify potentially inappropriate medications and potential errors of omissions in older patients.[101]

The concept of STOPP and START was originally designed to compensate for some of the flaws of the original Beers list. Beers 2012 emulated STOPP and START to some degree, but the ease of using and "sifting" through STOPP and START have made it a tool that is frankly, simpler to use and simpler to understand.

The total number of STOPP/START criteria increased by 31% from version 1 to version 2 between 2008 and 2013. Each criterion is accompanied by a concise explanation as to why the drug is included. This chapter will focus on the most important. The list printed below reflects the medications the United States has access to. Given that, this list is a derivation of what is published in the original STOPP/START.

The panel consisted of 19 experts from 13 countries in Europe, who are recognized for their expertise in geriatric medicine and pharmacotherapy in older people. They created STOPP and START to capture common and important instances of inappropriate prescribing and organized it by physiological systems. They also paid special attention to drugs affecting fall risk and opiate use in elders. Finally, they included medications that improve outcomes and quality of life as well. It was a unique and appropriate way of looking at medications to be discontinued in geriatric adults as well as those that should be used in geriatric adults.

STOPP AND THE CARDIOVASCULAR SYSTEM

- Digoxin for heart failure with preserved systolic ventricular function (no clear evidence of benefit).

- Verapamil or diltiazem with NYHA Class III or IV heart failure (may worsen heart failure).

- Use of a beta-blocker in combination with verapamil as it may cause heart block.

- Beta blocker with symptomatic bradycardia (< 50/min), type II heart block or complete heart block (risk of profound hypotension, asystole).

- Amiodarone as first-line antiarrhythmic therapy in supraventricular tachyarrhythmias; it has a higher risk of side-effects than beta-blockers, digoxin, verapamil or diltiazem.

- Loop diuretic for dependent ankle edema without clinical, biochemical or radiological evidence of heart failure, liver failure, nephrotic syndrome or renal failure.

  – no evidence of efficacy, leg elevation and /or compression hosiery.

- Loop diuretic as first-line monotherapy for hypertension (lack of outcome data for this indication; safer, more effective alternatives available).

- Loop diuretic for treatment of hypertension with concurrent urinary incontinence (may exacerbate incontinence).

- Thiazide diuretic with current significant hypokalemia (i.e. serum K+ < 3.0 mEq/L), hyponatremia (i.e. serum Na+ < 130 mEql/L), hypercalcemia (i.e. corrected serum calcium > 10.6 mg/dL), or with a history of gout (since gout can be precipitated by thiazide diuretics).

- Centrally-acting antihypertensives (e.g., methyldopa, clonidine, guanfacine), unless clear intolerance of, or lack of efficacy with, other classes of antihypertensives.

- ACE inhibitors or angiotensin receptor blockers (ARBs) in patients with hyperkalemia.

- Aldosterone antagonists such as spironolactone (Aldactone®) or eplerenone (Inspra®) with concurrent potassium-sparing drugs (e.g. ACEIs, ARBs, amiloride, triamterene) without monitoring of serum potassium (risk of dangerous hyperkalemia; i.e., > 6.0 mEq/L – serum potassium should be monitored regularly; i.e., at least every 6 months).

- Phosphodiesterase type-5 inhibitors such as sildenafil (Viagra®), tadalafil (Cialis®), or vardenafil (Levitra®) in severe heart failure characterized by hypotension; i.e., systolic BP < 90 mmHg, or concurrent daily nitrate therapy for angina (risk of cardiovascular collapse).

In general, medications with narrow therapeutic ranges should be used cautiously in older adults since renal function tends to affect the outcomes of these medications. Digoxin is one such medication and is also listed in the Beers criteria. In older adults, digoxin for heart failure with preserved systolic ventricular function has not shown any clear evidence of benefit and should be avoided. This is of even more importance in the presence of renal insufficiency or an acute kidney injury (AKI).

All providers learn about the risks associated with using beta-blockers in patients with a history of chronic obstructive pulmonary disease (COPD). There is a small risk of bronchospasm associated with their use but COPD exacerbation has been shown to be associated with a 3.5-fold increase in the rate of acute myocardial infarction (AMI) compared to those without COPD.[102] Consequently, beta-blockers (BB) are indeed appropriate for patients with COPD; however, clinicians should use selective beta-blockers (nebivolol, metoprolol) rather than non-selective beta-blockers (carvedilol, propranolol) due to this small risk of bronchospasm.

Any beta-blocker used in the presence of older adults with a heart rate < 50/min or used in combination with verapamil or diltiazem in type II or complete heart block risks complete heart block or asystole; the two should be avoided in combination.

Amiodarone, as is noted in the Beers Criteria, should be avoided as a first-line antiarrhythmic as a consequence of higher-risk side-effects that can occur.

Loop diuretics increase the risk of dehydration for any patient, but in the old and frail this is of particular importance. Loop diuretics used for dependent ankle edema without any clinical signs of heart failure has not been proven to be efficacious, but has also been shown to increase the risk of an acute kidney injury. In addition, loop diuretics should not be used as first-line monotherapy for hypertension.

Thiazide diuretics (hydrochlorothiazide, chlorthalidone) have long been known to exacerbate gout and should be avoided in patients with this history, but they can also lower blood sodium levels as well as blood potassium levels.

Centrally acting antihypertensives pose significant risk for falls, as is also noted in the Beers Criteria.

STOPP AND ANTIPLATELET/ANTICOAGULANT DRUGS

- Long-term aspirin at doses greater than 160mg per day (increased risk of bleeding, no evidence for increased efficacy).

- Aspirin with a past history of peptic ulcer disease without concomitant PPI (risk of recurrent peptic ulcer).

- Aspirin, clopidogrel, dipyridamole, vitamin K antagonists, direct thrombin inhibitors or factor Xa inhibitors with concurrent significant bleeding risk, (i.e., uncontrolled severe hypertension, bleeding diathesis, recent non-trivial spontaneous bleeding).

  – high risk of bleeding

- Aspirin plus clopidogrel as secondary stroke prevention, unless the patient has a coronary stent(s) inserted in the previous 12 months or concurrent acute coronary syndrome or has a high grade symptomatic carotid arterial stenosis (no evidence of added benefit over clopidogrel monotherapy).

- Aspirin in combination with vitamin K antagonist, direct thrombin inhibitor or factor Xa inhibitors in patients with chronic atrial fibrillation without a clear indication for aspirin.

  – no added benefit from aspirin

- Antiplatelet agents with vitamin K antagonist, direct thrombin inhibitor or factor Xa inhibitors in patients with stable coronary, cerebrovascular or peripheral arterial disease.

  – no added benefit from dual therapy

- Ticlopidine in any circumstances since clopidogrel (Plavix®) and prasugrel (Effient®) have similar efficacy, stronger evidence and fewer side-effects.

- Vitamin K antagonist, direct thrombin inhibitor or factor Xa inhibitors for first deep venous thrombosis without continuing provoking risk factors (e.g., thrombophilia) for > 6 months, since there is no proven added benefit.

- Vitamin K antagonist, direct thrombin inhibitor or factor Xa inhibitors for first pulmonary embolus without continuing provoking risk factors (e.g., thrombophilia) for > 12 months, since there is no proven added benefit.

- NSAID and vitamin K antagonist, direct thrombin inhibitor or factor Xa inhibitors in combination (risk of major gastrointestinal bleeding).
- NSAID with concurrent antiplatelet agent(s) without PPI prophylaxis (increased risk of peptic ulcer disease).

Aspirin inherently increases the risk of GI hemorrhage, especially as the dose is increased or if it's used in the presence of other NSAIDs.[103] In STOPP/START, long-term aspirin use at a dose >160mg per day is not recommended. In the United States, doses are to be kept ≤ 100 mg/d[104] except in some special circumstances involving stents. In general, if a patient has a history of peptic ulcer disease (PUD) and is on aspirin, then an H_2-antagonist or preferably a proton-pump inhibitor (PPI) should be prescribed concomitantly for safety. Additionally, aspirin, clopidogrel, dipyridamole, vitamin K antagonists, direct thrombin inhibitors or factor Xa inhibitors with concurrent significant bleeding risk (i.e., uncontrolled severe hypertension, bleeding diathesis, recent non-trivial spontaneous bleeding) pose a very high risk of bleeding and risk and benefits need to be weighed. Even in secondary stroke prevention, aspirin plus clopidogrel has not shown added benefit over clopidogrel monotherapy unless the patient has a coronary stent(s) inserted in the previous 12 months or concurrent acute coronary syndrome or has a high grade symptomatic carotid arterial stenosis. Furthermore, aspirin in combination with vitamin K antagonist, direct thrombin inhibitor or factor Xa inhibitors in patients with chronic atrial fibrillation is no longer recommended due to no added benefit from one agent alone.

In STOPP/START, antiplatelet agents with vitamin K antagonists, direct thrombin inhibitors or factor Xa inhibitors in patients with stable coronary, cerebrovascular or peripheral arterial disease have shown to have no added benefit from dual therapy and is not encouraged.

Ticlopidine (Ticlid®) was added to the 2014 STOPP/START criteria, given that clopidogrel (Plavix®) and prasugrel (Effient®) have similar efficacy, stronger evidence and fewer side-effects.

Vitamin K antagonists, direct thrombin inhibitors or factor Xa inhibitors carry with them bleeding risk. There is no proven added benefit for first uncomplicated deep venous thrombosis (DVT) without continuing provoking risk factors (e.g., thrombophilia) for greater than 6 months because the risk of a life-threatening hemorrhage outweighs the benefit it provides. Furthermore, these same agents for a first uncomplicated pulmonary embolus for longer than 12 months' duration is not warranted and should be discontinued as well.

As was noted in the Beers Criteria, NSAIDs and vitamin K antagonists, direct thrombin inhibitors or factor Xa inhibitors, and antiplatelet agents carry with them a major risk of GI bleeding. The risks and benefits clearly need to be weighed in the presence of these medications.

STOPP and the Central Nervous System

- Tricyclic antidepressants (TCAs) with dementia (risk of worsening cognitive impairment), TCAs with glaucoma (likely to exacerbate glaucoma).
- TCAs with cardiac conductive abnormalities (pro-arrhythmic effects).
- TCAs with prior history of urinary retention (likely to worsen retention).

> Note: all benzodiazepines should be withdrawn gradually if taken for more than 4 weeks as there is a risk of causing a benzodiazepine withdrawal syndrome if stopped abruptly.

- TCAs with prostatism or prior history of urinary retention (risk of urinary retention).
- Initiation of TCAs as first-line antidepressant treatment due to a higher risk of adverse drug reactions with TCAs than with SSRIs or SNRIs.
- Neuroleptics with moderate-marked antimuscarinic/anticholinergic effects such as chlorpromazine (Thorazine®), clozapine (Clozaril®), or fluphenazine (Prolixin) with a history of prostatism or previous urinary retention due to the high risk of urinary retention.
- Selective serotonin re-uptake inhibitors (SSRIs) with a history of clinically significant current or recent hyponatremia < 130 mEql/L.
- Benzodiazepines for ≥ 4 weeks (no indication for longer treatment; risk of prolonged sedation, confusion, impaired balance, falls, and traffic accidents).
- Antipsychotics other than quetiapine (Seroquel®) or clozapine (Clozaril) in those with parkinsonism or Lewy Body disease due to the risk of severe extra-pyramidal symptoms.
- Anticholinergics/antimuscarinics to treat extra-pyramidal side-effects of neuroleptic medications due to the risk of anticholinergic toxicity.

- Anticholinergics/antimuscarinics in patients with delirium or dementia
  – risk of exacerbation of cognitive impairment.
- Neuroleptic antipsychotic in patients with behavioral and psychological symptoms of dementia (BPSD) unless symptoms are severe and other non-pharmacological treatments have failed (increased risk of stroke).
- Neuroleptics as hypnotics, unless sleep disorder is due to psychosis or dementia (risk of confusion, hypotension, extra-pyramidal side effects, and falls).
- Acetylcholinesterase inhibitors with a known history of persistent bradycardia (< 60 beats/min.), heart block or recurrent unexplained syncope or concurrent treatment with drugs that reduce heart rate such as beta-blockers, digoxin, diltiazem, verapamil (risk of cardiac conduction failure, syncope and injury).
- Phenothiazines as first-line treatment, since safer and more efficacious alternatives exist (phenothiazines are sedating, have significant anti-muscarinic toxicity in older people, with the exception of prochlorperazine for nausea/vomiting/vertigo and chlorpromazine for relief of hiccoughs).
- Levodopa or dopamine agonists for benign essential tremor.
- First-generation antihistamines since safer, less toxic antihistamines are now widely available.

As has been mentioned earlier (see Chapter 7), tricyclic antidepressants (TCAs) are risky when used in geriatric adults. They are strongly anticholinergic medications and therefore will worsen cognition, worsen symptoms associated with glaucoma, are known to cause cardiac conduction abnormalities, and worsen urinary retention. Given that, SSRIs and SNRIs are considerably safer and these agents should be considered over TCAs. Even so, that needs to be weighed against the risk of hyponatremia. The reported incidence of SSRI-associated hyponatremia has been variable, ranging from 0.5% to 32%, and was most often observed in older adults.[105] In general, SSRIs with a history of clinically significant current or recent hyponatremia less than 130 mEql/L should be considered unsafe since they increase the risk of delirium, falls and lethargy.

Neuroleptic agents – more commonly known as first-generation or "typical" antipsychotics, especially those with moderate or marked antimuscarinic/anticholinergic effects – chlorpromazine (Thorazine), clozapine (Clozaril®), or fluphenazine (Prolixin®) – should be avoided due to the high risk of urinary retention in patients with a history of prostatism or previous urinary retention. In the United States, medications like haloperidol (Haldol®) and thioridazine (Mellaril®) would also be included. These medications also risk extrapyramidal symptoms (EPS) and have little evidence for efficacy given the risk except for those on palliative or hospice care.

There is little place for the use of benzodiazepines for longer than 4 weeks. Evidence lacks, since side effects – prolonged sedation, confusion, impaired balance, falls, and traffic accidents – outweigh benefits in many circumstances. Benzodiazepines are also known to be habit-forming but discontinuance or withdrawal of these medications should be gradual if taken for more than 4 weeks as there is a risk of causing a benzodiazepine withdrawal syndrome if stopped abruptly including causing seizures.

As a general rule, avoid antipsychotics other than quetiapine (Seroquel®) or clozapine (Clozaril) in patients with Parkinson's or dementia with Lewy Body, or those with parkinsonism, since those agents risk severe extra-pyramidal symptoms (EPS). Furthermore, prescribing cascades should be avoided, such as the addition of anticholinergics/antimuscarinics to treat extra-pyramidal side-effects of neuroleptic medications since they risk anticholinergic toxicity or worsen delirium or dementia.

First- and second-generation neuroleptic antipsychotics, such as those described in Chapter 7, should be avoided, especially in those patients with behavioral and psychological symptoms of dementia (BPSD), unless symptoms are severe and other non-pharmacological treatments have failed. In addition, neuroleptics as hypnotics should be avoided due to the high risk of confusion, hypotension, extra-pyramidal side effects, and falls unless the sleep disorder is due to psychosis.

Acetylcholinesterase inhibitors (Aricept®, Exelon®, Razadyne®) should be avoided in patients with a known history of persistent bradycardia (< 60 beats/min.), heart block or recurrent unexplained syncope or concurrent treatment with drugs that reduce heart rate such as beta-blockers, digoxin, diltiazem, and verapamil which can risk cardiac conduction failure thereby increasing the risk of syncope and injury.

Phenothiazines – including the antiemetic promethazine (Phenergan®) – can be sedating and have significant anti-muscarinic toxicity in older people. Exceptions include prochlorperazine (Compazine®) for nausea, vomiting or vertigo and chlorpromazine (Thorazine®) for relief of hiccoughs.

Levodopa or dopamine agonists for benign essential tremor should be avoided since there is no evidence of efficacy.

Finally, first-generation antihistamines, as noted in the "Top 10 Dangerous Drugs" (Chapter 10) should be avoided. Safer, less toxic antihistamines are now widely available.

STOPP AND THE RENAL SYSTEM

- Digoxin at a long-term dose greater than 125μg/day if eGFR < 30 ml/min/1.73m^2 as it can risk digoxin toxicity especially if plasma levels not measured.
- Direct thrombin inhibitors such as dabigatran (Pradaxa®) if eGFR < 30 ml/min/1.73m^2 due to the risk of bleeding.
- Factor Xa inhibitors such as rivaroxaban (Xarelto®), apixaban (Eliquis®), or edoxaban (Savaysa®) if eGFR < 15 ml/min/1.73m^2 secondary to risk of bleeding.
- NSAIDs if eGFR < 50 ml/min/1.73m^2 due to significant risk of deterioration in renal function.
- Colchicine if eGFR < 10 ml/min/1.73m^2 due to significant risk of deterioration in renal function.
- Metformin if eGFR < 30 ml/min/1.73m^2 as it may risk lactic acidosis.

The following drugs (above) are potentially inappropriate in older people with acute or chronic kidney disease with renal function below particular levels of eGFR. They include digoxin, direct thrombin inhibitors, factor Xa inhibitors, NSAIDs, colchicine and metformin. Until recently in the United States, metformin was not prescribed for certain level of creatinine clearance or eGFR. In April 2016, these guidelines were changed and the Food and Drug Administration (FDA) suggested that the metformin labeling would now reflect this new information and provide specific recommendations on the drug's use in patients with mild to moderate kidney impairment. They also recommending avoiding creatinine guidelines and focusing on eGFR instead.[106]

STOPP AND THE GASTROINTESTINAL SYSTEM

- Prochlorperazine or metoclopramide with Parkinsonism secondary to risk of exacerbating Parkinsonian symptoms.

- PPI for uncomplicated peptic ulcer disease or erosive peptic esophagitis at full therapeutic dosage for > 8 weeks; dose reduction or earlier discontinuation indicated.
- Drugs likely to cause constipation (e.g. antimuscarinic/anticholinergic drugs, oral iron, opioids, verapamil, aluminum antacids) in patients with chronic constipation where non-constipating alternatives are available.
- Oral elemental iron doses greater than 200 mg daily (e.g., ferrous fumarate> 600 mg/day, ferrous sulfate > 600 mg/day, ferrous gluconate > 1800 mg/ day; no evidence of enhanced iron absorption above these doses).

Prochlorperazine (Compazine®) or metoclopramide (Reglan®) with Parkinson's disease or parkinsonism may exacerbate parkinsonian symptoms. As is newly noted in the 2015 Beers Criteria, STOPP/START have made this recommendation since well before the Beers Criteria was published. The use of proton-pump inhibitors (PPIs) for peptic ulcer disease (PUD) is a mainstay treatment. However, treatment longer than 8 weeks in patients that are asymptomatic is not indicated.

Furthermore, drugs that are likely to cause constipation, such as antimuscarinic or anticholinergic drugs, oral iron (especially in high dose), opioids, verapamil, and aluminum antacids, are to be avoided since they can clearly worsen constipation. It should also be noted that for those patients taking elemental iron, there is no added benefit to doses greater than 200mg/ day and some studies have suggested that death rates are higher for those taking iron chronically.[107]

STOPP AND THE RESPIRATORY SYSTEM

- Theophylline as monotherapy for COPD. There are safer, more effective alternatives; risk of adverse effects due to narrow therapeutic index.
  – this tends to be more frequent in Europe.
- Systemic corticosteroids instead of inhaled corticosteroids for maintenance therapy in moderate-severe COPD (unnecessary exposure to long-term side-effects of systemic steroids and more effective inhaled therapies are available).
- Anti-muscarinic bronchodilators such as ipratropium with glaucoma can worsen glaucoma – or cause bladder outflow obstruction which may worsen urinary retention.

- Benzodiazepines with acute or chronic respiratory failure; i.e., $pO_2 < 60$ $\pm$ $pCO_2 > 50$ as they can risk exacerbation of respiratory failure.

Theophylline as a monotherapy for COPD is not indicated, especially considering there are more effective alternatives available. In addition, and as has been stated before, any medication that has a narrow therapeutic window, such as theophylline, must be used cautiously in older adults

Inhaled corticosteroids are preferred agents over systemic corticosteroids in moderate-severe COPD. The long-term side-effects of systemic steroids include GI hemorrhage, diabetes mellitus, glaucoma, osteoporosis, edema and hypertension.

Narrow angle glaucoma (a serious eye condition that may cause loss of vision), may worsen and become an acute end-angle glaucoma with the use of nebulized ipratropium. It may also worsen urinary retention.

Lastly, unless a patient is on palliative or hospice care, benzodiazepines should be avoided with acute or chronic respiratory failure since they can risk exacerbation of respiratory failure.

STOPP AND THE MUSCULOSKELETAL SYSTEM

- Non-COX-2 selective non-steroidal anti-inflammatory drugs (NSAIDs) with history of peptic ulcer disease or gastrointestinal bleeding, unless with concurrent histamine H_2-receptor antagonist or PPI (risk of peptic ulcer relapse).
- NSAIDs with established hypertension as they risk exacerbation of hypertension.
- NSAIDs with heart failure as they risk exacerbation of heart failure.
- Long-term use of NSAIDs (>3 months) for relief of osteoarthritis pain where acetaminophen has not been tried; simple analgesics preferable and usually as effective for pain relief.
- Long-term corticosteroids (>3 months) as monotherapy for rheumatoid arthritis due to risk of major systemic corticosteroid side-effects.
- Corticosteroids (other than periodic intra-articular injections for mono-articular pain) for osteoarthritis (risk of systemic corticosteroid side-effects).
- Long-term NSAID or colchicine for prevention of relapses of gout where there is no contraindication to a xanthine-oxidase inhibitor, such as allopurinol (Zyloprim®) or febuxostat (Uloric®) since these are the first choice prophylactic drugs in gout.

- COX-2 selective NSAIDs with concurrent cardiovascular disease (increased risk of myocardial infarction and stroke).
- NSAID with concurrent corticosteroids without PPI prophylaxis (increased risk of peptic ulcer disease).
- Oral bisphosphonates in patients with a history of upper gastrointestinal disease; i.e., dysphagia, esophagitis, gastritis, duodenitis, or peptic ulcer disease, or upper gastrointestinal bleeding.
  - risk of relapse/exacerbation of esophagitis, esophageal ulcer, esophageal stricture.

The risks associated with non-COX-2 selective non-steroidal anti-inflammatory drugs (NSAIDs) in older adults has long been known and have been discussed in detail throughout this book. In rare cases, older adults may require them to manage pain. In those rare circumstances, concurrent H_2-antagonists or proton-pump inhibitors (PPIs) should be prescribed to protect against present or future GI hemorrhage.

NSAIDs should be avoided in the presence of established hypertension or heart failure. Though NSAIDs may be warranted for short-term relief of pain in the treatment of gout, long-term management is not indicated unless there is a contraindication to xanthine-oxidase inhibitors (see below). Long-term use of NSAIDs (>3 months as noted by STOPP/START) where simple acetaminophen has not been tried or considered is contraindicated.

The World Health Organization (WHO) has an analgesic ladder that is usually preferred in geriatrics to NSAIDs for pain relief.[108] When possible medical personnel should attempt to follow the analgesic ladder for pain relief.

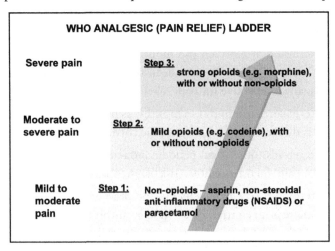

WHO ANALGESIC (PAIN RELIEF) LADDER

Severe pain — Step 3: strong opioids (e.g. morphine), with or without non-opioids

Moderate to severe pain — Step 2: Mild opioids (e.g. codeine), with or without non-opioids

Mild to moderate pain — Step 1: Non-opioids – aspirin, non-steroidal anit-inflammatory drugs (NSAIDS) or paracetamol

Figure 9.1: WHO Analgesic Ladder

Furthermore, a handful of patients may use systemic corticosteroids as monotherapy for rheumatoid arthritis and less commonly osteoarthritis. Unless these corticosteroids are used for periodic intra-articular injections, prolonged use of these agents carry with it substantial risks that have been discussed throughout this book. Alternate agents or specialty referral should be considered.

COX-2 selective NSAIDs with concurrent cardiovascular disease should also be evaluated as a substantial risk since it can increase the risk of myocardial infarction and stroke.

Lastly, oral bisphosphonates in patients with a current or recent history of upper gastrointestinal disease – dysphagia, esophagitis, gastritis, duodenitis, or peptic ulcer disease, or upper gastrointestinal bleeding – have risks of relapse or worsening esophagitis, esophageal ulcer, and esophageal stricture.

STOPP AND THE UROGENITAL SYSTEM

- Bladder antimuscarinic drugs with dementia or cognitive impairment (risk of increased confusion, agitation).
- Bladder antimuscarinic drugs with narrow-angle glaucoma (risk of acute exacerbation of glaucoma).
- Bladder antimuscarinic drugs with chronic prostatism (risk of urinary retention). Alpha$_1$-blockers in those with symptomatic orthostatic hypotension or micturition syncope (risk of precipitating recurrent syncope).

Bladder antimuscarinic drugs include a large class of medications that worsen dementia or mild-cognitive impairment and can also exacerbate behaviors associated with dementia. They also risk acute exacerbation of glaucoma, worsen constipation, and increase the likelihood of urinary retention. Agents in this class including tolterodine (Detrol or Detrol LA®), oxybutinin (Ditropan, Ditropan XL, Oxytrol®), darifenacin (Enablex®), trospium (Sanctura or Sanctura XR®), fesoterodine (Toviaz®), flavoxate (Urispas®) and solifenacin (Vesicare®) should be avoided.

Alpha$_1$-blockers, as was discussed in the Beers Criteria, increase the risk of symptomatic orthostatic hypotension or syncope while urinating. The risk of precipitating recurrent syncope is high and therefore should be avoided.

STOPP AND THE ENDOCRINE SYSTEM

- Sulfonylureas with a long duration of action, such as chlorpropamide (Diabinese®), glimepiride (Amaryl®) with type 2 diabetes mellitus secondary to the high risk of hypoglycemia.

- Thiazolidenediones such as rosiglitazone (Avandia®), pioglitazone (Actos®) in patients with heart failure since it risks exacerbation of heart failure.

- Beta-blockers in those with diabetes mellitus and frequent hypoglycemic episodes due to the risk of suppressing hypoglycemic symptoms.

- Estrogens with a history of breast cancer or venous thromboembolism (increased risk of recurrence). Oral estrogens without progesterone in patients with intact uterus (risk of endometrial cancer).

- Androgens (male sex hormones) in the absence of primary or secondary hypogonadism risk androgen toxicity without any proven benefit outside of the hypogonadism indication.

Chlorpropamide (Diabinese®) and glimepiride (Amaryl®) are long-acting secretagogues that stimulate pancreatic islet beta cells to release insulin. The half-life of these medications is extraordinarily long. These islet cells are indifferent to producing insulin even when an older adult stops eating, has nausea leading to anorexia or diarrhea or vomiting. Consequently, the risk of hypoglycemia is increased and enhanced with these long-acting agents.

Beta-blockers, when used in diabetics may lead to a decreased risk of myocardial infarction. However, for those patients who are "brittle" and whose sugars rise and fall very quickly, beta-blockers have been known to "mask" hypoglycemia and consequently lead to the risk of an adverse drug event. Patients who are at risk of hypoglycemia should have beta-blockers discontinued.

The Women's Health Initiative and the HERS trials demonstrated the risk of prolonged use of estrogens (see Chapter 7). Estrogen alone with a history of breast cancer or venous thromboembolism (VTE) carries a risk of recurrence. Likewise, estrogens without progesterone should be avoided in patients with an intact uterus who risk endometrial cancer.

Lastly, male sex hormones have taken on new meaning with the commercialization of "low T" as a condition needing to be treated. In the absence of primary or secondary hypogonadism, which endocrinology can assess for, there is no proven benefit of testosterone replacement.

STOPP THOSE DRUGS THAT INCREASE THE RISK OF FALLS

- Benzodiazepines (sedative, may cause reduced sensorium, impair balance).
- Neuroleptic drugs (may cause gait dyspraxia or parkinsonism).
- Vasodilator drugs known to cause hypotension in those with persistent postural hypotension; i.e., alpha$_1$-receptor blockers, calcium channel blockers, long-acting nitrates, ACE inhibitors, angiotensin I receptor blockers, with persistent postural hypotension (recurrent drop in systolic blood pressure ≥ 20mmHg) risks syncope and falls.
- Hypnotic Z-drugs such as eszopiclone (Lunesta®), zolpidem (Ambien®), zaleplon (Sonata®) may cause protracted daytime sedation and ataxia.

Anytime you hear the words fall or fracture listed in the same sentence as geriatric, the provider must consider the medication that is being prescribed or used. Benzodiazepines, neuroleptic agents that vasodilate the arterial tree (see above) can lead to falls and subsequent fractures. Additionally, the "hypnotics" traditionally used for sleep latency have been added to the STOPP Criteria.

STOPP AND ANALGESICS

- Use of oral or transdermal strong opioids (morphine, oxycodone, fentanyl, buprenorphine, methadone, tramadol, pentazocine) without following the WHO analgesic ladder is not indicated.
- Regular opiates (as distinct from PRN) without concomitant laxatives (risk of severe constipation).
- Long-acting opiates without short-acting opioids for break-through pain (risk of persistence of severe pain).

When it comes to pain the World Health Organization follows an "analgesic ladder" that is very specific; it is noted in Figure 9.1. Use of this ladder should be considered. Pain medications that are not titrated appropriately in older adults risk causing lethargy, fatigue, constipation and delirium. Long-term opioids without short-acting agents present for break-through risk persistence of severe pain.

STOPP AND ANTIMUSCARINIC/ANTICHOLINERGIC DRUG BURDEN

- Concomitant use of two or more drugs with antimuscarinic/anticholinergic properties (e.g. bladder antispasmodics, intestinal antispasmodics, tricyclic antidepressants, first-generation antihistamines) risks increased antimuscarinic/anticholinergic side-effects and should be avoided.

START (SCREENING TOOL TO ALERT TO RIGHT TREATMENT)

The biggest advantage of STOPP and START is the Screening Tool to Alert to Right Treatment. It is rare in geriatrics to find instances where medical providers evaluate how to improve both quality and quantity of life but START has accomplished that. Unless an older person's clinical status is end-of-life where the focus is more palliative than curative, the following drug therapies should be considered.

START AND THE CARDIOVASCULAR SYSTEM

- Vitamin K antagonists or direct thrombin inhibitors or factor Xa inhibitors in the presence of chronic atrial fibrillation.
- Aspirin (75 mg – 160 mg once daily) in the presence of chronic atrial fibrillation, where Vitamin K antagonists or direct thrombin inhibitors or factor Xa inhibitors are contraindicated.
- Antiplatelet therapy (aspirin or clopidogrel (Plavix®) or prasugrel (Effient®) or ticagrelor (Brilinta®) with a documented history of coronary, cerebral or peripheral vascular disease.
- Antihypertensive therapy where systolic blood pressure is consistently > 160 mmHg and/or diastolic blood pressure consistently >90 mmHg; if systolic blood pressure > 140 mmHg and/or diastolic blood pressure > 90 mmHg, if diabetic.
- Statin therapy with a documented history of coronary, cerebral or peripheral vascular disease, unless the patient's status is end-of-life or age is > 85 years.
- Angiotensin converting enzyme (ACE) inhibitor with systolic heart failure and/or documented coronary artery disease.
- Beta-blocker with ischemic heart disease.
- Appropriate beta-blocker such as bisoprolol (Zabeta®), nebivolol (Bystolic®), metoprolol (Toprol®) or carvedilol (Coreg®) with stable systolic heart failure.

Despite the risks associated with anticoagulants, they are still the standard of care for atrial fibrillation; the risk of stroke, in most circumstances, outweighs the risk associated with warfarin or Novel Oral Anti-Coagulants (NOACs). Where these agents are contraindicated however, low-dose aspirin is an acceptable choice. Make note that in the United States, aspirin <100mg is preferred in atrial fibrillation.

Aspirin, Plavix®, Effient®, or Brilinta® is indicated for those with a documented history of coronary artery disease (CAD), cerebrovascular disease (CVD) or peripheral vascular disease (PVD).

When systolic blood pressures are greater than 160 mmHg, treatment should be considered. The American Geriatrics Society recommends treatment to standards of the JNC-VIII[109], but when blood pressures run low in older adults or older adults are symptomatic (dizzy or lightheaded), it can increase the risk of falls. Unlike JNC-VIII guidelines, START recommended treatment levels to a different standard due to the risk of falls associated with having too low a blood pressure. JNC-VIII evaluated those same risks and adopted some – but not all – of those guidelines similar to what is noted in START.

Statins are medications that have substantial efficacy and with a documented history of coronary, cerebral or peripheral vascular disease they should be used. However, statins are best used when the patient's functional status remains independent for activities of daily living and life expectancy is greater than 5 years. Otherwise, statins may not be necessary for older adults. START recommends their use for patients whose status is not end-of-life or age is <85 years.

Angiotensin converting enzyme (ACE) inhibitors have substantial benefits in older adults. Some of the distinct advantages include their benefits for systolic heart failure and coronary artery disease.

Beta-blockers make the START criteria for patients with ischemic heart disease as well as heart failure, given that it's a beta-blocker that has been well studied and shown to be beneficial in systolic heart failure. Those medications include: bisoprolol (Zabeta®), nebivolol (Bystolic®), metoprolol (Toprol®) or carvedilol (Coreg®).

START AND THE RESPIRATORY SYSTEM

- Regular inhaled beta-2 agonist or antimuscarinic bronchodilators like ipratropium (Atrovent®) or tiotropium (Spiriva®) for mild to moderate asthma or COPD.

- Regular inhaled corticosteroid for moderate-severe asthma or COPD where FEV_1 is <50% of predicted value and repeated exacerbations require treatment with oral corticosteroids.

- Home continuous oxygen with documented chronic hypoxemia (i.e., pO_2 < 60 or SaO_2 < 89%).

Patients with mild-to-moderate COPD or asthma should START beta-2 agonist or inhaled anticholinergic agents. Additionally, inhaled (not to be confused with oral) corticosteroids for moderate-to-severe asthma or COPD as defined by the World Health Organization and GOLD standards should be **START**ed in older adults. Finally, for those older patients who are hypoxic, the clinician should START oxygen as it has been shown not only to improve outcomes data for older adults but also quality of life.

START and the Central Nervous & Ophthalmic Systems

- L-DOPA in idiopathic Parkinson's disease with definite functional impairment and resultant disability without orthostatic hypotension.

- Non-TCA (tricyclic antidepressant) drugs in the presence of persistent major depressive symptoms.

- Acetylcholinesterase inhibitors such as donepezil (Aricept®), rivastigmine (Exelon®) or galantamine (Razadyne®) for mild to moderate Alzheimer's dementia or Lewy Body dementia (DLB).

- Topical prostaglandin or beta-blocker for primary open-angle glaucoma.

- Selective serotonin reuptake inhibitor (or SNRI or pregabalin if SSRI contraindicated) for persistent severe anxiety that interferes with independent functioning.

- Dopamine agonist such as ropinirole (Requip®) or pramipexole (Mirapex®) or rotigotine transdermal (Neupro®) for restless legs syndrome (RLS), once iron deficiency anemia and severe renal failure have been excluded.

In the newest version of START, several new recommendations are present in the central nervous system. L-DOPA for patients with Parkinson's disease in the absence of orthostatic hypotension improves functional impairment and disability associated with the disease. Eventually these drugs will lack efficacy, but initially Parkinson's patients get significant relief of symptoms and functional benefits as well.

Other included agents are non-TCA (non-tricyclic antidepressants) in the presence of persistent major depressive symptoms. Acetylcholinesterase inhibitors were also recommended in both Alzheimer's and DLB for the benefits they can provide both functionally and behaviorally. These too eventually become less efficient but early on in the course of disease, both of these medications palliate signs and symptoms associated with a very debilitating decline.

An additional recommendation includes the use of SSRIs, SNRIs or pregabalin for persistent severe anxiety if it interferes with independent functioning; gabapentin, which acts similarly to pregabalin, can also be helpful.[110]

Lastly, for those suspected of having RLS, dopamine agonists – ropinirole (Requip®) or pramipexole (Mirapex®) or rotigotine (Neupro®) – have shown to be effective. It is important to make sure that renal failure or iron deficiency anemia has been ruled out.

START AND THE GASTROINTESTINAL SYSTEM

- Proton pump inhibitor with severe GERD or peptic strictures requiring dilatation.
- Fiber supplement for chronic, symptomatic diverticular disease with constipation.

In the GI system, the use of PPIs with severe reflux or peptic strictures requiring dilatation should be utilized and continued. For practical purposes START also recommends fiber supplementation for those patients with chronic, symptomatic diverticular disease in the presence of constipation.

START AND THE MUSCULOSKELETAL SYSTEM

- Disease-modifying anti-rheumatic drugs (DMARDs) with active disabling rheumatoid disease. Bisphosphonates and vitamin D and calcium in patients taking long-term systemic corticosteroid therapy. Vitamin D and calcium supplements in patients with known osteoporosis and/or previous fragility fracture(s) and/or bone mineral density T-scores > –2.5 in multiple sites. Bone anti-resorptive or anabolic therapy such as bisphosphonates, teriparatide (Forteo®), denosumab (Prolia® or Xgeva®) in patients with documented osteoporosis, where no pharmacological or clinical status contraindication exists. DXA T-scores > -2.5 in multiple sites and/or previous history of fragility fracture(s). Vitamin D supplement in older people who are housebound or experiencing falls or with osteopenia.

Xanthine-oxidase inhibitors such as allopurinol (Zyloprim®) or febuxostat (Uloric®) with a history of recurrent episodes of gout. Folic acid supplement in patients taking methotrexate.

The musculoskeletal system is widely affected in geriatric adults. It is therefore recommended for patients with rheumatoid disease, that DMARDs (disease-modifying anti-rheumatic drugs) be initiated. It is best to do this with the guidance of a rheumatologist. Should the patient be taking methotrexate, folic acid should be added.

Bisphosphonates and vitamin D should also be considered in older adults using oral corticosteroids. Bisphosphonates are risky in older adults once their GFR is <50mL/min/1.73m^2 so caution should be exercised in patients fitting this profile.

In patients with T-scores > –2.5, anabolic or resorptive therapy is recommended unless a pharmacological contraindication exists. It should also be noted that multiple sites should be involved and/or previous history of fragility fractures noted. Vitamin D supplementation should be given if older adults are known to be falling and osteopenic.

Lastly, patients with recurrent episodes of gout should have allopurinol (Zyloprim®) or febuxostat (Uloric®) added to minimize recurrence.

START AND THE ENDOCRINE SYSTEM

- ACE inhibitor or angiotensin receptor blocker (if intolerant of ACE inhibitor) in diabetes with evidence of renal disease; i.e., dipstick proteinuria or microalbuminuria >30mg/24 hours with or without serum biochemical renal impairment.

In the endocrine system, ACE inhibitors or angiotensin receptor blockers (ARBs) are medications that provide benefit in diabetes with nephropathy. It is important to START these agents, notwithstanding any contraindications, in this circumstance.

START AND THE UROGENITAL SYSTEM

- Alpha$_1$-receptor blockers with symptomatic prostatism, where prostatectomy is not considered necessary.
- 5-alpha reductase inhibitors with symptomatic prostatism, where prostatectomy is not considered necessary.
- Topical vaginal estrogen or vaginal estrogen pessary for symptomatic atrophic vaginitis.

For patients with symptomatic prostatism, where prostatectomy is not considered necessary, alpha$_1$-receptor blockers – tamsulosin (Flomax®), silodosin (Rapaflo®) – or 5-alpha reductase inhibitors – dutasteride (Avodart®), finasteride (Proscar®) – or both – dutasteride/tumsuolosin (Jalyn®) – are clinically indicated.

For women who may complain of urinary incontinence, seen often in atrophic vaginitis, vaginal estrogens – estradiol cream (Estrace®) – may be appropriate.

START AND THE ANALGESICS

- High-potency opioids in moderate-severe pain, where acetaminophen or low-potency opioids are not appropriate to the pain severity or have been ineffective.
- Laxatives in patients receiving opioids regularly.

For geriatric adults in pain, high-potency opioids may be indicated. It should be noted that these medications are oftentimes used when acetaminophen, or low-potency opioids have been ineffective and the WHO Analgesic Ladder (Figure 9.1) has been trialed.

Additionally, laxatives should be prescribed for patient receiving opioids regularly to minimize risk of constipation

START AND VACCINES

- Seasonal trivalent influenza vaccine annually.
- Pneumococcal vaccine at least once after age 65 according to national guidelines.

A welcome addition to the START guidelines is the seasonal trivalent influenza vaccine. Influenza is an aggressive killer of older adults. In the 2014-2015 seasons, >90% of influenza deaths occurred among persons ≥65 years of age and rates of influenza-associated hospitalizations among people 65 and older were much higher than in previous years. In that seasonal period, there were an estimated 8.3 million illnesses, 4.7 million medical visits and 758,000 flu hospitalizations.[111] And, although the incidence of influenza can vary widely between years, approximately 36,000 deaths are directly associated with influenza every year in the United States.[112] The great flu pandemic of 2009-2010 is estimated to have taken between 106,000 to nearly 400,000 people.[113] GET VACCINATED! Especially if you are elderly.

An additional vaccine is the pneumococcal vaccine (PPSV23) which requires vaccination at least once after the age of 65 years of age. Another vaccine, recently introduced in the United States is the pneumococcal conjugate vaccine (PCV13). It is currently recommended for all adults 65 years or older as well.

Adults aged ≥65 years who have not previously received the pneumococcal vaccine or whose previous vaccination history is unknown should receive a dose of PCV13 first, followed by a dose of PPSV23 approximately one year later. For those adults who have already received PPSV23, a single dose of PCV13 should be given approximately one year later.[114]

CHAPTER 10

The Top 10 Dangerous Drugs

If Mark Beers taught us one thing of value, it's that older adults are underserved. They are given medications many times out of convenience, or guidelines, and in reality, there are very few guidelines that academically demonstrate benefit for the "old-old" (85 and greater). It's something this author likes to call "extrapolative medicine." There are no studies that apply to this age-bracket, so instead, clinicians extrapolate from young patients to our older patients. It's a very dangerous way to practice medicine, yet many clinicians just turn a blind eye.

The real art of medicine is bringing it all together and that is why older adults should, at the very least, have a consultation with a geriatric internist.

The "Top Ten List" was developed with older adults in mind. The American Geriatrics Society Foundation for Health in Aging created this list so that older people could be conscious of medications, including those available over-the-counter, that can be purchased without a prescription. They also recommended that medical personnel post and distribute the list in clinics so that older adults could read it and question why a medication was placed on the list. Finally, it recommended that if you are an older adult, and if you are taking any of these medications, that you should talk to your healthcare provider or pharmacist.

Medication(s)	➡	Reason(s)

Medication(s)	Reason(s)
Non-Steroidal Anti-Inflammatory Drugs (NSAIDs) - Used to reduce pain & inflammation **AVOID NSAIDs** like indomethacin (Indocin®), piroxicam (Feldene®), ibuprofen (Advil®, Motrin®) and salsalate (Disalcid®). If you take NSAIDs regularly, and have a history of ulcers **OR** are 75 or older, you may need to protect your stomach against bleeding with a prescription medication. Since these drugs increase the risk of bleeding, don't use NSAIDs together with aspirin, clopidogrel (Plavix®), dabigatran (Pradaxa®), rivaroxaban (Xarelto®), edoxaban (Savaysa®), apixaban (Eliquis®), dipyridamole (Persantine®), prasugrel (Effient®), ticlopidine (Ticlid®), or warfarin (Coumadin®).	**NSAIDs can increase the risk of indigestion, ulcers, and bleeding in your stomach or colon. They can also increase blood pressure, affect your kidneys, and make heart failure worse.**
AVOID digoxin (Lanoxin®) in doses greater than 0.125 mg. Digoxin is used to treat heart failure and irregular heartbeats.	**It can be toxic in older adults and people whose kidneys do not work well.**
AVOID Certain Diabetes Drugs as Glyburide (Diabeta®, Micronase®), glimerperide (Amaryl®) and chlorpropamide (Diabinese®).	**These can cause severe low blood sugar.**
AVOID Muscle Relaxants such as cyclobenzaprine (Flexeril®), methocarbamol (Robaxin®), and carisoprodol (Soma®), and similar medications	**They can leave you feeling groggy, confused, increase your risk of falls, cause constipation, dry mouth, and problems urinating. Plus, there is little evidence that they work well.**
AVOID Certain Medications used for Anxiety and/or Insomnia such as benzodiazepines, such as diazepam (Valium®), alprazolam (Xanax®), lorazepam (Ativan®), clonazepam (Klonipin®) or chlordiazepoxide (Librium®). Sleeping pills such as eszopiclone (Lunesta®), zaleplon (Sonata®) and zolpidem (Ambien®).	**They can increase your risk of falls, fractures, confusion and amnesia.**

Medication(s)	➡	Reason(s)

Medication(s)	Reason(s)
AVOID Certain Anticholinergic Drugs Antidepressants such as amitriptyline (Elavil®) and imipramine (Tofranil®), anti-Parkinson drugs trihexyphenidyl (Artane®) and benztropine (Cogentin®). Irritable bowel syndrome drugs similar to dicyclomine (Bentyl®). Overactive bladder drug similar to oxybutynin (Ditropan®).	**They can cause confusion, constipation, problems urinating (especially in men), blurry vision, and low blood pressure.**
AVOID the Pain Reliever meperidine (Demerol)	**It can cause seizures/ confusion.**
AVOID Certain Over-the-Counter Products, AVOID products that contain the antihistamines diphenhydramine (Benadryl®) and chlorpheniramine (AllerChlor®, Chlor-Trimeton®) especially in men with prostate issues. AVOID over-the-counter sleep products, similar to Tylenol PM, Aleve PM, and Ibuprofen PM, which contain diphenhydramine. If you hear the word "PM" in a medication, it probably contains these products.	**Although these medications are sold without a prescription, they are not risk free. They can cause confusion, blurred vision, constipation, problems urinating, and dry mouth.**
If you are NOT being treated for psychosis, AVOID using Antipsychotics such as haloperidol (Haldol®), risperidone (Risperdal®), olanzapine (Zyprexa®) or quetiapine (Seroquel®).	**They can increase the risk of stroke or even <u>death</u>. They can also cause tremors, other side effects, as well as risk of falls.**
AVOID Estrogen pills and patches typically prescribed for hot flashes and other menopause-related symptoms.	**They can increase your risk of breast cancer, blood clots, and even dementia.**

Figure 10.1: Top 10 Medications Geriatric Adults Should Avoid

At this point, many of you will realize this list is redundant. All of the medications on this list have been discussed at one point or another in this book. Feel free to copy Figure 10.1 and distribute it, so that older adults can be educated about the risks of medications that many times they can get readily over the counter.

Ten Medications Older Adults Should Avoid or Use with Caution[115]

(1) **Non-Steroidal Anti-Inflammatory Drugs (NSAIDs) which are oftentimes used to reduce pain and inflammation**

Recommendation:

AVOID NSAIDs like indomethacin (Indocin®), piroxicam (Feldene®), ibuprofen (Advil®, Motrin®) and salsalate (Disalcid®).

If you take NSAIDs regularly, and have a history of ulcers or are 75 years of age or older, you may need to protect your stomach against bleeding with a prescription medication such as misoprostol (Cytotec) or a proton pump inhibitor such as omeprazole (Prilosec).

Because of the increased risk of bleeding, don't use NSAIDs together with aspirin, clopidogrel (Plavix®), dabigatran (Pradaxa®), rivaroxaban (Xarelto®), edoxaban (Savaysa®), apixaban (Eliquis®), dipyridamole (Persantine®), prasugrel (Effient®), ticlopidine (Ticlid®), or warfarin (Coumadin®).

Reason:

NSAIDs can increase the risk of indigestion, ulcers, and bleeding in your stomach or colon. They can also increase blood pressure, affect your kidneys, and make heart failure worse.

OOOOO

(2) **AVOID digoxin (Lanoxin) in doses greater than 0.125 mg (125mcg) which are oftentimes used to treat heart failure and irregular heartbeats.**

Recommendation:

AVOID digoxin in doses higher than 0.125mg or 125mcg as studies have not shown benefit.

Reason:

It can be toxic in older adults and people whose kidneys do not work well.

OOOOO

③ AVOID Certain Diabetes Drugs

Recommendation:

AVOID medications like glyburide (Diabeta®, Micronase®), glimepiride (Amaryl®) and chlorpropamide (Diabinese®). They stay in the body for long periods of time and are difficult to excrete out of the body from the kidney.

Reason:

These can cause severe low blood sugar.

OOOOO

④ AVOID Muscle Relaxants

Recommendation:

AVOID medications like cyclobenzaprine (Flexeril®), methocarbamol (Robaxin®), and carisoprodol (Soma®), and similar medications. They are difficult to metabolize and they interact with other medications easily.

Reason:

They can leave you feeling groggy and confused, increase your risk of falls, and cause constipation, dry mouth, and problems urinating. Plus, there is little evidence that they work well.

OOOOO

⑤ AVOID Certain Medications used for Anxiety and/or Insomnia

Recommendation:

AVOID benzodiazepines, such as diazepam (Valium®), alprazolam (Xanax®), lorazepam (Ativan®), clonazepam (Klonipin®) or chlordiazepoxide (Librium®). Four of these medications have been linked to permanent memory loss or dementia.

AVOID sleeping pills such as eszopiclone (Lunesta®), zaleplon (Sonata®) and zolpidem (Ambien®).

Reason:

They can increase your risk of falls, fractures, motor vehicle accidents, and dementia as well as cause confusion. Because it takes your body a long time to get rid of these drugs, you could feel groggy and sleepy for a long time.

OOOOO

⑥ AVOID Anticholinergic Drugs

Recommendation:

AVOID antidepressants such amitriptyline (Elavil®) and imipramine (Tofranil®)

AVOID the anti-Parkinson drugs trihexyphenidyl (Artane®) and benztropine (Cogentin®)

AVOID irritable bowel syndrome drugs similar to dicyclomine (Bentyl®)

AVOID overactive bladder drugs similar to oxybutynin (Ditropan®)

Reason:

They can cause confusion, constipation, problems urinating, blurry vision, and low blood pressure. Men with an enlarged prostate should be particularly cautious because it can prevent them from urinating.

OOOOO

⑦ AVOID the pain reliever meperidine (Demerol®)

Recommendation:

AVOID this pain reliever

Reason:

It can increase the risk of seizures and can cause confusion.

OOOOO

⑧ AVOID Certain Over-the-Counter Products

Recommendation:

AVOID products that contain the antihistamines diphenhydramine (Benadryl®) and chlorpheniramine (AllerChlor®, Chlor-Trimeton®) particularly in men with an enlarged prostate because it can prevent them from urinating.

AVOID over-the-counter sleep products, similar to Tylenol PM, Aleve PM, and Ibuprofen PM, which contain diphenhydramine. If you hear the word "PM" in a medication, it probably contains these products.

Reason:

Although these medications are sold without a prescription, they are not risk free. Quite the contrary in fact! They can cause confusion, blurred vision, constipation, problems urinating, and dry mouth.

OOOOO

(9) **If you are NOT being treated for psychosis, AVOID using Antipsychotics**

Recommendation:

AVOID medications such as haloperidol (Haldol®), risperidone (Risperdal®), olanzapine (Zyprexa®) or quetiapine (Seroquel®).

Reason:

They can increase the risk of stroke or even death. They can also cause tremors and other side effects, as well as increase the risk of falls.

OOOOO

(10) **AVOID Estrogen pills and patches that are typically prescribed for hot flashes**

Recommendation:

AVOID these medications; though they can typically be prescribed for a short period of time to manage hot flashes and other menopause-related symptoms, in time they can cause a lot of harm.

Reason:

Studies demonstrate they can increase your risk of breast cancer, blood clots, and even dementia.

CHAPTER 11

The Controversy Surrounding Multivitamins and Other Medications

Multivitamin or mineral supplements account for almost one-sixth of all purchases of dietary supplements in the United States, worth an estimated total of $36.7 billion in 2014.[116] Overall, women are more likely to take multivitamins and minerals than men, and currently about half of adults report using 1 or more dietary supplements.[117]

IS YOUR MULTIVITAMIN KILLING YOU?

Recently, studies have been done to determine the safety of taking multivitamins and mineral supplements. These studies have also been reproduced[114,115] which attests to their reliability. One of the most important studies is the Iowa Women's Health Study which evaluated the use of vitamin and mineral supplements in relation to total mortality. A total of 38,772 women (mean age 61.6) were included in this analysis over 19 years. The results, STUNNING!

In multivariable adjusted proportional hazards regression models, the use of multivitamins was associated with increased risk of total DEATH when compared with corresponding nonuse. Total absolute risk increased by 2.4%, vitamin B6 (pyridoxine) increased the risk by 4.1%, folic acid 5.9%, iron by 3.9%, magnesium by 3.6%, zinc by 3.0% and copper by 18%. In fact, one of the only elements that didn't cause an increase in death was calcium, which was inversely related with an absolute risk reduction of 3.8%.[118,119]

Novel Oral Anti-Coagulants and Warfarin. Should I call 1-800-BAD-DRUG?

Warfarin, which was approved by the FDA in 1954, remains the most widely prescribed oral anticoagulant in the world for preventing thrombosis and thromboembolic disorders. Even so, warfarin has many concerns, including the need for regular monitoring, extensive drug–drug and drug–food interactions, and a delayed onset and long duration of action.

In 2010, the FDA approved the first novel oral anticoagulant (NOAC), dabigatran (Pradaxa®) and since that time, three more NOACs have come to market—rivaroxaban (Xarelto®), apixaban (Eliquis®), and edoxaban (Savaysa®). These newer agents offer monitoring-free options for preventing thrombosis, a fast onset of action (approximately 2-4 h vs. 48-72 h for warfarin) and a short half-life (approximately 5-17 h versus about 40 h for warfarin). In contrast to warfarin, NOACs have fewer drug interactions, which warrants less regular monitoring.

Until recently, the NOACs did not have specific reversal agents for bleeding complications; now these exist. For minor bleeding however, holding doses of the medication may be sufficient given the short half-lives in comparison to warfarin. For major bleeding, hemodynamic support may have been needed. Despite these differences, many clinicians were skeptical and prescriptions remained stagnant.

The data has now shown us the impact of these medications regarding efficacy and risk. The study this author chose was for ONLY elderly adults.

The study consisted of ten randomized-controlled trials that included 25,031 elderly participants. In the studies, they evaluated the risk of major or clinically relevant bleeding and showed that it was not significantly different between NOACs and conventional therapy in elderly adults. For the atrial fibrillation trials, NOACs were more effective than conventional therapy in prevention of stroke or systemic embolism. In trials involving deep vein thromboembolisms (VTE) or blood clots, NOACs also had a significantly lower risk of blood clots or VTE-related death than conventional therapy in elderly adults. Analysis for individual NOACs showed that the NOAC was noninferior or more effective than conventional therapy for efficacy and safety outcomes.[120]

Recommendations Regarding Vitamin D

As many as half of older adults in the United States with hip fractures are considered vitamin D deficient.[121] Cochrane analysis has shown that treatment with vitamin D_3 and calcium in weak, elderly, institutionalized individuals reduced the risk of fractures.[122]

In supplements and fortified foods, vitamin D is available in two forms, D_2 (ergocalciferol) and D_3 (cholecalciferol) that differ chemically only in their side-chain structure. And, while most geriatricians will give D_3 because of the purported absorptive benefits, evidence is unclear as to whether vitamin D_2 or D_3 is better. The NIH has given no firm evidence that any one agent is better than the other.

The American Geriatric Society has received some criticism for the concentration of serum vitamin D they target. A concentration of 30ng/mL (75nmol/L) is the minimum goal to achieve in older adults[123] according to their guidelines while other agencies have targeted higher levels suggesting morbidity outcomes may be better.[124] Regardless, nearly all studies suggest benefit with vitamin D.

RECOMMENDATIONS REGARDING VITAMIN E

Previous evidence suggested that oxidative stress was important in the pathogenesis of Alzheimer's disease. Consequently, a placebo-controlled, clinical trial of vitamin E in patients with moderately advanced Alzheimer's disease was conducted by the Alzheimer's Disease Cooperative Study. Subjects were treated with 2000 IU of vitamin E, and outcomes suggested that high dose vitamin E may slow functional deterioration.[125]

Years later however, suggestions were made that high dose vitamin E was causing higher rates of heart attacks so meta-analysis was done on dose-response relationships between vitamin E supplementation and total mortality. The conclusion: high-dose (≥400 IU/d) vitamin E supplements increased all-cause mortality and should be avoided.[126]

HOW MUCH SALT IS TOO MUCH? IS IT ONE SIZE FITS ALL?

Sodium is an essential nutrient yet numerous studies have shown that a high dietary salt intake increases blood pressure and risks increased cardiovascular and cerebrovascular events. This has generally been believed since increasing sodium intake is also associated with increasing blood pressure – a common risk factor in heart attack and stroke.

One of the best known diets – the DASH (Dietary Approaches to Stop Hypertension) diet – was designed to help treat or prevent high blood pressure and it includes, amongst other dietary recommendations, a low dietary salt intake of less than 2300mg, or lower, per day.[127]

Recently, there have been some suggestions that the data we were being "fed" – pun intended – was inaccurate. While low sodium intake (<2.0 g/d) has been achieved in many short-term clinical trials, sustained low sodium intake has not been achieved by any of the longer term clinical trials (>6-month duration). Consequently, prospective cohort studies were reviewed on more than 300,000 people, and suggested that the lowest risk of cardiovascular events and death occurs in populations consuming an average sodium intake range of 3–5 g/d. It also suggested that increased risk of cardiovascular events was associated with a sodium intake of >5 g/d.[128]

Pending further research, current evidence would suggest a recommendation for moderate sodium intake in the general population (3–5 g/d), with targeting the lower end of the moderate range among those with hypertension.

CHAPTER 12

Safely Prescribing Opioids

It is well known that as people age, pain becomes increasingly more common. Studies indicate that both community-dwelling older people and nursing home residents report pain on a nearly daily basis.[129, 130]

There are often medical, social and psychological, comorbidities that may contribute to pain and, in combination, they impact treatment response to it. Additionally, there is the risk of what may happen to an older person if doses are uptitrated too quickly or the patient has a reaction to pain medications.

Pain has long been known to contribute to declines in function which in turn accelerate the fragility that geriatricians see in the elderly.[131] Persistent pain has been shown to be associated with impaired physical function, increased risk of falls, sleep disruption, depression, anxiety, agitation, delirium and cognitive decline. Consequently, it is important for medical providers to approach pain in the older adult focusing on the older adult first and the patient with pain second. The basic principles of geriatric medicine usually suggest that pathology can make a patient vulnerable to stressors. Centering the treatment targets around those stressors may often lead to better outcomes than managing only the pathology itself.[132]

As an example, a patient with osteoarthritis may likely have degenerative disease that affects mobility. Consequently, the more important treatment target may be a co-existent depression and physical and occupational therapy to assist in mobility tactics.

Prescribing effective treatment starts with an accurate and comprehensive history and physical and highlights those comorbities that contribute to pain; e.g., depression and anxiety.

The main goal in the treatment of persistent pain is to maximize function and quality of life. To do this, a provider must consider the adverse effects that may be associated with treatment. And, due to the multifaceted nature of persistent pain, total pain elimination may not be a realistic goal. It is therefore important to ensure the older adult understands a provider's expectations regarding optimal pain management:

- Persistent pain is multifactorial in cause and requires both pharmacologic and nonpharmacologic strategies
- Persistent pain is manageable but not curable

Furthermore, the increased potential for drug-drug and drug-disease interactions as well as adverse drug events must always be considered when prescribing in the elderly.

NONPHARMACOLOGIC TREATMENTS — Nonpharmacological approaches to the management of persistent pain have been shown to be beneficial, cost effective, have few side effects, and are void of adverse drug events.[133] They encompass a wide array of options: physical interventions include physical therapy, acupuncture, acupressure, massage, etc. Psychological interventions include cognitive-behavioral therapy, meditation, and patient education; they should be considered for all persistent pain conditions.

PHARMACOLOGIC TREATMENTS — Patients whose pain is not diminished by nonpharmacological treatments should be considered for pharmacological therapy. In most cases, non-opioid medications are preferred over opioids for non-cancer pain. Analgesics should be initiated at the lowest effective dose, and titrated upward slowly to achieve pain control to minimize adverse effects. Medications used on a schedule rather than as needed are preferred for long-standing pain. Given that understanding, it is easy to see why frequent reassessment is needed in the elderly.

In some circumstances, localized use of injectable medications (e.g., joint injections, trigger point injections) may be preferred to systemic medications (e.g., oral analgesics). The choice of an appropriate initial agent is dependent upon a thorough evaluation of the cause of that pain: is it neuropathic versus nociceptive?

Non-opioid options

Acetaminophen — this is usually considered the first-line treatment in the management of mild persistent pain in the older adult because of its safety compared to other analgesics, particularly nonsteroidal anti-inflammatory drugs (NSAIDs) and opioids. The maximum safe dose in geriatric adults in 3 grams in 24 hours due to potential liver toxicity.[134] For patients who are frail, use multiple medications, or use alcohol on a regular basis, a maximum acetaminophen dose of 2 grams per day may be more appropriate.

Nonsteroidal anti-inflammatory drugs — In general, nonsteroidal anti-inflammatory drugs (NSAIDs) should be avoided and are not preferred in older adults; they are associated with a multitude of risk factors. If they are used, medical personnel should ensure the pain is nociceptive rather than neuropathic. Nociceptive pain is pain that results from damage to body tissue and usually described as a sharp, aching, or throbbing pain. After this determination is made, the lowest dose should be used and risk factors considered. Doses should be kept low and the choice of drug should be tailored to the patient's risk factors for gastrointestinal and cardiovascular disease. Naproxen may be a more reasonable choice in patients at risk of cardiovascular disease. Celecoxib (Celebrex®) may be a more reasonable choice in patients at risk of gastrointestinal hemorrhage.[135] The use of a proton pump inhibitor or misoprostol reduces but does not eliminate this risk, while use of systemic corticosteroids, anticoagulants, or antiplatelet agents increases this risk.

Additionally, a 2014 meta-analysis of 280 trials of NSAIDs versus placebo and 474 trials comparing NSAIDs, evaluated the risk for coronary and vascular events. COX-2 inhibitors (celecoxib), high-dose diclofenac and possibly ibuprofen increased this risk while naproxen did not appear to increase this risk.[136]

Topical and injected analgesics - Topical analgesics have the advantage of rarely causing systemic adverse effects, and may be a good option in the older patient. Injection therapy (e.g., joint injections, trigger point injections) should be considered where evidence supports its use.

Antidepressants - Antidepressants used in the treatment of chronic neuropathic pain include selective serotonin reuptake inhibitors (SSRIs), selective norepinephrine reuptake inhibitors (SNRIs), and tricyclic antidepressants (TCAs). All have side effects which may limit their use in geriatric adults.

TCAs are highly anticholinergic and those effects are heightened in older adults. The anticholinergic effects tend to also be more prominent with older TCAs (e.g., amitriptyline) than with newer TCAs (e.g., nortriptyline). They are all on the Beers Criteria!

SSRIs and SNRIs may be used in the treatment of persistent neuropathic pain and tend to have fewer cardiovascular and anticholinergic adverse effects than TCAs. Duloxetine (Cymbalta®) is an SNRI with an indication for chronic pain.[137] Both SSRIs and SNRIs may be associated with a higher fall risk in older adults.[138]

It is not widely known that tramadol (Ultram®) has effects similar to SSRIs and SNRIs. Tramadol produces anti-inflammatory actions similar to antidepressants because it also inhibits NE and 5HT reuptake. Dual action antidepressants mirtazapine (Remeron®), duloxetine (Cymbalta), and most notably venlafaxine (Effexor®), are chemically similar in structure to tramadol. However, extreme caution should be exercised in older adults using tramadol with a seizure disorder due to the potential risk for exacerbating a seizure whereas that same risk does not exist in those using SNRIs.

Anticonvulsants — Pregabalin (Lyrica®) and gabapentin (Neurontin®) have been shown to be effective in the treatment of neuropathic pain,[139,140] but this doesn't make them absent of side effects. The most common side effects are dizziness, somnolence, fatigue, and fluid retention.[141] For trigeminal neuralgia, carbamazepine (or possibly oxcarbazepine) is the treatment of choice but also risks hyponatremia.[142]

Muscle relaxants — Muscle relaxants are risky in older adults due to side effects. Many of the agents are included in the Beers Criteria and many lack efficacy altogether.

Opioid options—

Choosing a desirable opioid is not a simple task. Clinicians should consider the desired route of administration (e.g., sublingual, oral, or topical), the onset of action, the duration of action, interactions with other medications, coexisting medical conditions, and potency that could lead to undesirable side effects. In general, reasonable choices in older adults include oxycodone, hydrocodone, morphine, hydromorphone, fentanyl, buprenorphine, and methadone.

The majority of patients with chronic pain will use oral medications. Patients with difficulty swallowing may benefit from medications available in a liquid form (e.g., oxycodone, hydromorphone, morphine) or a transdermal patch (e.g., fentanyl, buprenorphine). For transdermal delivery methods, it should be noted that older adults have decreased subcutaneous tissue, and therefore absorption of these agents may ineffective. In general, all long-acting opioids should be avoided in opioid-naive patients, though patients with frequent or continuous daily pain may benefit from long-acting medications and for those with breakthrough pain, shorter-acting, immediate-release medications should be made available.

Renally cleared drugs (e.g., hydromorphone, morphine, oxycodone) should be reduced or non-renally cleared drugs (e.g., buprenorphine, fentanyl) selected when renal function is compromised in older adults. Even though there is no "rule" about dosing of opioids, a reasonable approach is to decrease the "usual" dose by 50 percent unless GFR > 60 mL/min/1.73m^2, and slowly titrate upwards until effective.

Risk/Benefits to Opioid Selection—

- Oxycodone is oftentimes used because of its shorter half-life, the absence of toxic metabolites, and availability in both the short- and long-acting forms.

- Hydrocodone is used because of its shorter half-life and for those who react poorly to oxycodone. It should be noted that the active metabolite for hydrocodone is hydromorphone so hydrocodone should be titrated slowly.

- Morphine has relatively few age-related changes in pharmacokinetics. Because increased sensitivity is common in the elderly, initial doses should be reduced. Active metabolites are cleared renally, so for those who are not acutely impaired, morphine should be avoided in patients with a GFR <30 mL/min/1.73m^2.[143]

- Hydromorphone is a short-acting medication and should be used primarily as a breakthrough medication. It should be used cautiously in older adults because of risks of delirium.

- Fentanyl is useful in patients with mild-moderate renal and hepatic dysfunction. It is a short-acting medication in oral or lozenge form but is also available as a transdermal patch.

- Buprenorphine is a high-affinity partial mu-opioid receptor agonist that is safer in renally-impaired patients. It comes in a sublinguinal formulation but special medical training is required prior to being allowed to administer this medication. One distinct advantage is the incidence of nausea, vomiting, and constipation are lower than with morphine.[144]

More problematic options in older adults include methadone. Methadone acts on both the mu-opioid receptor and the NMDA receptor. It has a very complicated pharmacokinetic and pharmacodynamic profile. Accordingly, methadone should only be initiated by clinicians who are familiar with its administration, long and variable half-life, and the risk of delirium associated with use.

Codeine is a weak analgesic that is metabolized to morphine in the liver. It has a higher incidence of nausea, vomiting than other opioids and due to the genetic differences amongst patients, it may be ineffective in patients of Asian and African descent.[145]

Mixed agonist/antagonist drugs (e. g., pentazocine) have higher rates of side effects with poor efficacy compared with other opioids.

Meperidine is to be avoided due to a toxic metabolite that can cause neurotoxicity/seizures; it is on the Beers Criteria.

Adverse effects of opioids encompass the central nervous system, the gastrointestinal system, and the respiratory system.

- The Central Nervous System — Opioid therapy can cause somnolence or clouding of the memory. In some patients it waxes and wanes, while in others it may persist. Caution should always be exercised since delirium equates to higher rates of mortality.[146]

- Balance — Use of opioids can lead to balance dysregulation and has been show to increase fall risk.[147]

- Recommendations from the American Geriatric Society suggest educating older adults about the risk of falls before opioids are prescribed and that balance and mobility are evaluated at baseline and through the course of treatment.

- Constipation — Constipation is the most common side effect of opioid therapy in older adults, and it can occur with any dose and with any duration of use. It is not only prudent but also wise medical practice to begin prophylactic laxative therapy when opioid treatment is initiated.

- Other gastrointestinal issues — Dry mouth and nausea are also common side effects of opioids. Gradual upward titration of the opioid dose is helpful.

- Respiratory — Respiratory depression, albeit a concern, is rare with the "start low, go slow" model of geriatrics. A more common associated risk is a sleep disorder, such as daytime somnolence.

For those patients with dementia, patient reliability can often be affected. Medical providers are challenged to determine if the pain being reported is from true pain-related suffering, perseveration, or a signal of some other type of distress such as anxiety associated with unfamiliar surroundings. Clinicians managing demented adults should not exclude the possibility of pain simply because of dementia which compromises any direct ability to communicate clearly at times. There is a plethora of rigorous scientific data on cognitive impairment and the impact on poor pain perception which can lead to undesirable behaviors.[148,149]

A model of thought for those with dementia suspected of having pain should include—

- A prescription of scheduled analgesics
- A stepped-care approach to analgesic prescribing
- Start low and go slow
- Monitor the patient as the clinician balances risks and benefits of pain treatment.

Adequate pain control may take the form of improvements in behavior and function. A randomized, double-blind, placebo-controlled, crossover trial demonstrated that social interactions and well-being were improved in nursing home residents with moderate-to-severe dementia with the administration of acetaminophen alone, at doses of 3 grams per day during a four-week period.[150] However, if no improvement is noted in function or behavior or overall benefit is not perceived, discontinue those medications and monitor.

Finally, the American Geriatrics Society has developed clinical practice guidelines for the Pharmacological Management of Persistent Pain in Older Persons for review.[151] It can be found here:

http://www.centralhealthline.ca/healthlibrary_docs/painMgmt_for_Older_Persons.pdf[152]

This review defines appropriate ways to consider pain management in the elderly.

CHAPTER 13

Practical Guidelines for Prescribers

As a general rule of thumb, appropriate prescribing in the elderly starts by using drug doses that are less likely to cause harm to elderly adults. In the United States, most studies just aren't done on the elderly and consequently, practitioners may start older adults on medication doses that would be appropriate for younger but not older adults. Furthermore, especially when speaking about the "old, old" (85 years or older), high medication doses can really be dangerous.

The list that follows includes practical guidelines for safe prescribing in the elderly adult:

- Consider non-pharmacological agents for treatment.
- Avoid prescribing prior to having a high index of suspicion for a diagnosis.
- Start low and go slow.
- Document the indication for each new drug that is started (to avoid using unnecessary drugs and to serve as reminder why the drug was chosen).
- Adjust doses for renal and hepatic impairment in the elderly.
- Avoid initiating two agents at the same time.
- Reach "target" doses before switching or adding additional agents (understand $t_{1/2}$).
- Document the risk of therapy versus its benefit.
- Choose the safest possible alternative (e.g., choosing Tylenol for arthritis over an NSAID).

- Check for potential drug-disease and drug-drug interactions.
- Avoid the "prescribing cascade" by ruling out that any new symptom(s) aren't the consequence of an existing drug.
- Attempt to prescribe a drug that will treat more than one existing problem.
- Determine therapeutic endpoints and most important, document it. If the therapeutic endpoint is not achieved as a consequence of the drug either having a side-effect or not working, discontinue the medication.
- Explain why the drug is being taken and educate patients about common adverse effects of each drug.
- Employ pharmacists as "reviewers" of medications.

As noted above, doses of medications in older adults, should generally be lower than that of their young counterparts. Starting doses of about one-third to one-half the usual non-geriatric adult dose is recommended. Once the drug is shown to be working, this can be followed by upward titration, when and where appropriate, until there is a desired effect. Uptitration frequency is dictated by a concrete understanding of a medication's half-life and a patient's renal clearance. Since *steady state* is not achieved for 5-6 half-lives, practitioners should evaluate for adverse effects before dosing or frequency of administration is adjusted.

It is particularly important to reconsider medication appropriateness and more importantly continuously evaluate this at subsequent visits. A model for appropriate prescribing for older patients is shown in Figure 13.1. The process considers the life expectancy and the quality of life measures in reviewing the need for existing medications and in making new prescribing decisions. As an example, if a patient's life expectancy is short and the goals of care are more palliative in approach, then prescribing a medication to prevent heart disease may require several years to realize any benefit; it may not be considered appropriate. This is most evident when patients have severe dementia.[153]

Much attention has been paid to overprescribing for older adults, but under-prescribing appropriate medications is also of concern. One study of older adults in a VA outpatient population with a mean age of 75 years found that underuse of appropriate medications occurred as much as 64% of the time.[155] Despite this, it should also be pointed out that "under-prescribing" may be prevalent as a consequence of a clinician's informed decisions to "underprescribe" in order to improve compliance with essential medications while limiting drug interactions, minimizing risk, and improving impact on quality of life. As an example, a patient with diabetes might be recommended to be on an anti-glycemic agent (or two), beta-blocker, ACE inhibitor, aspirin, and statin. In this context, the risk for a drug-drug interaction doubles if one additional medication is added (see Chapter 5).

APPROPRIATE PRESCRIBING IN THE ELDERLY[154]

(1) Is there an indication for the drug?

(2) Is the medication effective for the condition?

(3) Is the dosage correct?

(4) Are the directions correct?

(5) Are the directions practical?

(6) Are there clinically significant drug-disease interactions?

(7) Are there clinically significant drug-disease/condition interactions?

(8) Is there unnecessary duplication with other drugs?

(9) Is the duration of therapy acceptable?

(10) Is this drug the least expensive alternative compared with others of equal usefulness?

Figure 13.1: Appropriate Prescribing in the Elderly

A STEPWISE APPROACH TO PRESCRIBING

When it is deemed necessary to prescribe, there are certain steps medical professionals should follow and abide by:

(1) **Review and re-review current drug therapy** — Periodic, but continuous, evaluation of a patient's drug regimen is an essential component in caring for the elderly. As such, a review of medications (approximately annually for clinic patients and once every 3 months for patients in assisted living and long-term care facilities) may result in positive changes to or even discontinuation of prescribed drug therapy. Changes may include discontinuing a therapy (as needed or routine) prescribed for either an acute situation or an indication that no longer exists. It may also include substituting a therapy with a potentially safer agent, a change in drug dosage, or adding a new more appropriate

medication. Furthermore, medication reviews should include a consideration whether an acute or chronic change in patient condition might necessitate dosing adjustment, whether there is a potential for a drug-drug interaction, a drug side-effect, or whether the current drug regimen could be decreased.

Furthermore, at least once annually (or after a hospitalization), encourage patients to bring all (EVERYTHING) of the bottles or pills they are using or HAVE USED in the past year; it's best to ask them to empty their "medicine cabinet" and bring those medications in. Patients may not consider over-the-counter products, ointments, vitamins, eye drops, or herbal medicines to be drug therapies. Make sure to mention that the visit will be only to review medications and nothing else.

(2) **Discontinue unnecessary therapy** — Appropriately, clinicians may feel reluctant to stop certain medications, especially if the patient seems to be tolerating the therapy and the treatment was initiated by another clinician. A common example is digoxin, which has many drug-drug interactions, risks digoxin toxicity in the elderly and has variable efficacy in older adults. Despite that it does have some benefit in heart failure and atrial fibrillation.

The decision to discontinue a medication is determined in part by the goals of care for that patient and the risks of adverse effects for that patient. Approaches to assessing whether a drug is truly necessary for a given patient are presented throughout this book. Furthermore, some preventive and other therapies may no longer be beneficial to patients with shorter-than-expected life spans.

It is reasonable to taper off most medications so as to minimize withdrawal reactions, and to allow symptom monitoring, unless dangerous signs or symptoms indicate a need for abrupt medication withdrawal. Certain common drugs require tapering, including beta blockers, opioids, barbiturates, clonidine, gabapentin, and antidepressants. In general, the appropriateness of any therapy should be reconsidered when other medical conditions develop that impact a patient's long-term prognosis, unless the therapies are thought to increase comfort or the patient and/ or family desire it.

(3) **Consider adverse drug events for any new symptom** — Before adding any new therapy to the patient's drug regimen, carefully consider whether a new medical condition could be linked to an existing drug therapy.

Clinicians should evaluate the drug regimen approximately 2 months prior to see if the symptom may be related to the drug therapy. In doing so, a prescribing cascade can be avoided.

④ ALWAYS **consider non-pharmacological approaches** — Some conditions in older adults may improve with simple lifestyle modification in lieu of pharmacotherapy. As an example, simple weight loss and reduced sodium intake, as shown in the Trial of Non-pharmacologic Interventions in the Elderly (TONE trial) allowed for discontinuation of antihypertensive medication in about 40% percent of the cases.[156]

⑤ **Substitute with safer alternatives** — When drug therapy is indicated for the older patient, it may be possible to substitute a safer alternative for the current regimen. As an example, the newer seizure agents (Lamictal® or Keppra®) have fewer drug-drug interactions and don't require blood monitoring.

⑥ **Reduce the dose** — Many adverse drug events are dose-related. When prescribing drug therapies, it is important to use the lowest dose needed to obtain a clinical benefit.

⑦ **Simplify the dosing schedule** — When multiple medications are taken, the complexity around it increases the likelihood of poor compliance or confusion with dosing. Studies indicate that once-daily medical regimens result in up to twice as many adherent days.[157]

⑧ **Utilize pharmacists** – Studies clearly show benefit when pharmacists conduct a review of medications. One study showed that medication change rates ranged from 46% to 68% in the presence of a pharmacist. This number improves to a striking 73% when physicians, care managers and participants/caregivers were all contacted by pharmacists.[158]

CHAPTER 14

An Algorithm to Discontinuing Medications

The Garfinkel method (see Figure 14.1), is an algorithm designed to feasibly and safely discontinue medications and address the issue of polypharmacy in the elderly.[159] As is seen in the algorithm, the provider starts by determining if an evidence-based consensus exists for the use of, and continuation of, the medication in question. If the practitioner can determine the medication in question is indicated at its current dose, considering the patient's age group and disability level, and the benefits outweigh the risk, then the medication should be continued. Otherwise, move to the next step in the algorithm.

This next step is to determine if the indication is valid and relevant given the patient's age and frailty. If the clinician answers no to this question, the drug should be stopped. However, if the indication appears relevant, the healthcare provider should then consider if the possible adverse reactions to the medication outweigh the benefits in a patient who is old and frail. If the adverse reactions outweigh the benefits, the drug should be discontinued by way of a taper if necessary.

If the clinician believes the medication continues to provide benefit, the next step would be to determine if there are any side effects from the medication. If the practitioner answers yes to the question, given they've already determined the necessity of the medication, then they should consider switching the medication to a safer alternative. However, if the answer is "no" then the professional should ask if there is another drug that may be superior to the one in question; i.e., cheaper alternative, more expensive but safer alternative. If another drug is superior, consider shifting to another drug. Should there be no superior agent, consider if the dose could be reduced and do so if no significant risk is present. Otherwise, the healthcare professional would continue with the same dose.

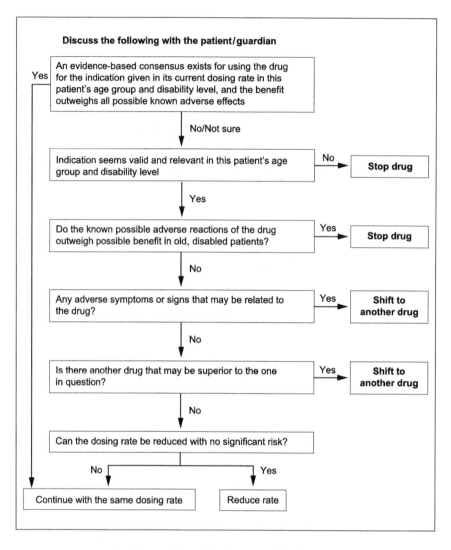

Figure 14.1: The Garfinkel Method

Dr. Garfinkel developed this algorithm by testing it on a cohort of 70 community-dwelling patients. Through its implementation, Dr. Garfinkel was able to discontinue 81% of the medications patients were taking. Incredibly, only 2% were restarted, and no significant adverse events were attributable to discontinuation over a 13-month follow-up.[160]

SUMMARY AND RECOMMENDATIONS

Never before have doctors had such an abundance of therapeutic medicinal options. And not surprisingly, the elderly consume more medications than ever before in history. Both pharmacokinetic and pharmacodynamic changes seen in this age group lead to increased plasma drug concentrations and increased drug sensitivity; aging influences every aspect of physiologic drug processing. As such, when evaluating older adults, the possibility of an adverse drug event (ADE) should <u>always</u> be considered. Additionally, new symptoms should be considered drug-related until proven otherwise.

Clinicians must be alert to drug-drug interactions, identifying medications that should not be prescribed, or those that should be prescribed with caution, and consider the individual patient.

A step-wise approach to prescribing for older adults should include: considering non-pharmacologic alternative strategies; periodic review of current drug therapy; discontinuing medications that may no longer be necessary; considering safer alternatives, using the appropriate dose, and including those medications that are beneficial to both outcomes and quality of life.

Since the elderly portion of the population is expanding more rapidly than any other, to recognize and prevent problems associated with medications is one of the most critical safety and economic issues facing the healthcare system today. Since this problem demands multidisciplinary involvement, everyone from families to practitioners can play a key role in making a difference.

References

1   US Census Bureau, Population Division 2012.

2   US Census Bureau, Population Division 2012.

3   Hanlon JT, Schmader KE, et al. Adverse drug events in high risk older outpatients. *J Am Geriatr Soc* 1997; 45:945–948.

4   Qiuping Gu et al. Prescription Drug Use Continues to Increase: US Prescription Drug Data for 2007-2008. *NCHS Data Brief* No. 42, September 2010.

5   Lazarou J, Pomeranz BH, Corey PN. Incidence of adverse drug reactions in hospitalized patients: a meta-analysis of prospective studies. *JAMA* 1998; 279:1200–5.

6   Qiuping Gu et al. Prescription Drug Use Continues to Increase: US Prescription Drug Data for 2007–2008. *NCHS Data Brief* No. 42, September 2010.

7   Jackson MG, Drechsler-Martell CR, Jackson EA. Family practice residents' prescribing patterns. *Drug Intell Clin Pharm.* 1985 Mar; 19(3):205–9.

8   Pleym H, Spigset O, et al. Gender differences in drug effects: implications for anesthesiologists. *Acta Anaesethsiol Scand* 2003; 47:241–259.

9   Petrone K, Katz P. Approaches to appropriate drug prescribing for the older adult. *Prim Care.* 2005 Sep; 32(3):755–75.

10   Corsonello A, Pedone C, et al. Concealed renal insufficiency and adverse drug reactions in elderly hospitalized patients. *Arch Intern Med.* 2005; 165:790–795.

11   National Kidney Foundation, 2002. Accessed online: http://www.kidney.org/professionals/kdoqi/guidelines_ckd/p5_lab_g4.htm. Last accessed 03/04/12.

12   Simon J et al. Interpreting the estimated glomerular filtration rate in primary care: Benefits and pitfalls. *Clev Clin J Med.* 2011; 78(3):189–195.

13   Smith GL et al. Renal impairment and outcomes in heart failure. Systematic review and meta-analysis. *J Am Coll Cardiol.* 2006; 47: 1987–1996.

14   Smith GL. Serum urea nitrogen, creatinine, and estimators of renal function. Mortality in older patients with cardiovascular disease. *Arch Intern Med.* 2006; 166: 1134–1142.

15   Shamseddin MK, Parfrey PS. Sudden cardiac death in chronic kidney disease: epidemiology and prevention. *Nat Rev Nephrol.* 2011 Mar; 7(3):145–54.

16   Smith GL et al. Renal impairment and outcomes in heart failure. Systematic review and meta-analysis. *J Am Coll Cardiol.* 2006; 47: 1987–1996.

[17]   Smith GL. Serum urea nitrogen, creatinine, and estimators of renal function. Mortality in older patients with cardiovascular disease. *Arch Intern Med.* 2006; 166: 1134–1142.

[18]   Schmucker DL. Liver function and phase I metabolism in the elderly: a paradox. *Drugs Aging* 2001; 18: 837–51.

[19]   Hornbrook MC, Stevens VJ, et al. Preventing falls among community–dwelling older persons: results from a randomized trial. *The Gerontologist* 1994:34(1):16–23.

[20]   Kiely DK, Jons RN, Bergmann MA et al. Association between psychomotor activity delirium subtypes and mortality amongst newly admitted post-acute facility patients. *J Gerontol A Biol Sci Med Sci.* 2007;62(2):174–179.

[21]   Adapted from: Pacala JT, Sullivan GM, eds. *Geriatrics Review Syllabus: A Core Curriculum in Geriatric Medicine.* 8th ed. New York: American Geriatrics Society; 2013.

[22]   Steinman MA, Landefeld CS, Rosenthal GE, et al. Polypharmacy and prescribing quality in older people. *J Am Geriatr Soc.* 2006; 54(10):1516.

[23]   Hamilton HJ, Gallagher PF et al. Inappropriate prescribing and adverse drug events in older people. *BMC Geriatrics* 2009; 9:5.

[24]   Lazarou J, Pomeranz BH, et al. Incidence of adverse drug reactions in hospitalized patients: a meta-analysis of prospective studies. *JAMA.* 1998; 279(15): 1200–1206.

[25]   FDA Adverse Events Reporting System (FAERS): FAERS Reporting by Patient Outcomes by Year. Accessed online: http://www.fda.gov/Drugs/GuidanceComplianceRegulatory Information/Surveillance/AdverseDrugEffects/ucm070461.htm Last accessed on: 11/8/2015.

[26]   Lazarou J, Pomeranz BH, et al. Incidence of adverse drug reactions in hospitalized patients: a meta-analysis of prospective studies. *JAMA.* 1998; 279(15): 1200–1206.

[27]   Budnitz DS, Lovegrove MC, Shehab N et al. Emergency hospitalizations for adverse drug events in older Americans. *N Engl J Med* 2011; 365:2002–2012.

[28]   Denham MJ. Adverse drug reactions. *Br Med Bull.* 1990; 46(1): 53–62.

[29]   Hanlon JT, Schmader KE, et al. Adverse drug events in high risk older outpatients. *J Am Geriatr Soc* 1997; 45:945–948.

[30]   Pacala JT, Sullivan GM, eds. *Geriatrics Review Syllabus: A Core Curriculum in Geriatric Medicine.* 8th ed. New York: American Geriatrics Society; 2013.

[31]   Clyne B, Smith S, et al. Effectiveness of a Multifaceted Intervention for Potentially Inappropriate Prescribing in Older Patients in Primary Care: A Cluster-Randomized Controlled Trial (OPTI-SCRIPT Study). *Ann Fam Med* 2015 13:510–511.

[32]   Adapted and used with the gracious permission of Professor Graham Davies Professor of Clinical Pharmacy & Therapeutics. Citing Website: Polypharmacy and Adverse Drug Reactions (ADR) in the Elderly. Last accessed online March 8, 2012 from http://www. docstoc.com/docs/77757229/Poly-pharmacy-and-Adverse-Drug-Reactions-in-the-Elderly.

[33]   Adapted from: Budnitz DS, Lovegrove MC, Shehab, Nadine S et al. Emergency Hospitalizations for Adverse Drug Events in Older Americans. *N Engl J Med* 2011; 365:2002–2012.

34 Budnitz DS, Lovegrove MC, Shehab, Nadine S et al. Emergency Hospitalizations for Adverse Drug Events in Older Americans. *N Engl J Med* 2011; 365:2002–2012.

35 Adapted from: Budnitz DS, Lovegrove MC, Shehab, Nadine S et al. Emergency Hospitalizations for Adverse Drug Events in Older Americans. *N Engl J Med* 2011; 365:2002–2012.

36 Gurwitz JH, Field TS, Avorn J, et al. Incidence and preventability of adverse drug events in nursing homes. *Am J Med* 2000;109(2):87–94.

37 Onder G, Vetrano DL, Cherubini A, et al. Prescription drug use among older adults in Italy: A country-wide perspective. *J Am Med Dir Assoc* 2014; 15:531. e11e531.e15.

38 Dwyer LL, Han B, Woodwell DA, Rechtsteiner EA. Polypharmacy in nursing home residents in the United States: Results of the 2004 National Nursing Home Survey. *Am J Geriatr Pharmacother* 2010; 8:63e72.

39 Hajjar ER, Cafiero AC, and Hanlon JT. Polypharmacy in elderly patients. *Am J Geriatr Pharmacother* 2007;5:345–351.

40 Coggins, MD. Focus on Adverse Drug Events. *Todays Geriatric Medicine* 2015; 8(6);8.

41 Rochon PA, Gurwitz JH. Optimizing drug treatment in elderly people: the prescribing cascade. *BMJ* 1997; 315:1097.

42 Jacob S, Spinler S. Hyponatremia with Selective Serotonin-Reuptake Inhibitors in Older Adults. *Ann Pharmacother* 2006; 40:1618–22.

43 *Mosby's Medical Dictionary*, 8th edition. 2009.

44 Citing website: New Molecular Entity Approvals for 2015. Retrieved November 20, 2015 from: http://www.fda.gov/Drugs/DevelopmentApprovalProcess/DrugInnovation/ucm430302.htm.

45 Citing website: FDA approved drugs. Retrieved November 20, 2012 from: http://www.centerwatch.com/drug-information/fda-approvals/default.aspx?DrugYear=2015.

46 Carrillo JA, Herraiz AG, Ramos SI et al. Role of the smoking-induced cytochrome P450 (CYP) 1A2 and polymorphic CYP2D6 in steady-state concentration of olanzapine. *J Clin Psychopharmacol.* 2003; 23:119–27.

47 Amir O, Hassan Y, et al. Incidence of risk factors for developing hyperkalemia when using ACE inhibitors in cardiovascular diseases. *Pharm World Sci.* 2009 Jun; 31(3):387–93.

48 Masclee GM, Valkhoff VE, Coloma PM et al. Risk of upper gastrointestinal bleeding from different drug combinations. *Gastroenterology.* 2014 Oct; 147(4):784–792.e9.

49 Lanas A, Scheiman J. Low-dose aspirin and upper gastrointestinal damage: epidemiology, prevention and treatment. *Curr Med Res Opin.* 2007; 23: 163–173.

50 Masclee GM, Valkhoff VE, Coloma PM et al. Risk of upper gastrointestinal bleeding from different drug combinations. *Gastroenterology.* 2014 Oct; 147(4):784–792.e9.

51 Masclee GM, Valkhoff VE, Coloma PM et al. Risk of upper gastrointestinal bleeding from different drug combinations. *Gastroenterology.* 2014 Oct; 147(4):784–792.e9.

[52] Savarese G, Rosano G, McMurray J et al. Efficacy and safety of novel oral anticoagulants in patients with atrial fibrillation and heart failure: A meta-analysis of phase III clinical trials. *J Am Coll Cardiol.* 2015; 65(10_S).

[53] Mehran R, Rao SV, Bhatt DL, et al. Standardized bleeding definitions for cardiovascular clinical trials: a consensus report from the bleeding academic research consortium. *Circulation.* 2011; 123(23):2736–47.

[54] Adapted from: Wadhera RK, Russell CE, Piazza G. Cardiology patient page. Warfarin Versus Novel Oral Anticoagulants: How to Choose? *Circulation.* 2014; 130: e191–e193.

[55] 2003 Beers Criteria as noted in Roehl B, Talati A, Parks S. Medication prescribing for older adults. *Ann Long-Term Care.* 2006 Jun; 14(6):33–9.

[56] The American Geriatrics Society 2012 Beers Criteria Update Expert Panel. American Geriatrics Society updated Beers criteria for potentially inappropriate medication use in older adults. *J Am Geriatr Soc* 2012; 60:616–31.

[57] American Geriatrics Society 2015 Updated Beers Criteria for Potentially Inappropriate Medication Use in Older Adults. *J Am Geriatr Soc.* 2015; 63(11):2227–2246.

[58] American Geriatrics Society 2015 Updated Beers Criteria for Potentially Inappropriate Medication Use in Older Adults. *J Am Geriatr Soc.* 2015; 63(11):2227–2246.

[59] Kahneman, D. (2011). *Thinking, Fast and Slow.* New York, NY: Farrar, Straus and Giroux.

[60] Porter RS. (2011) *The Merck Manual of Diagnosis and Therapy* Nineteenth Edition.

[61] Adapted from: Stone N, Ashraf M, et al. Surveillance Definitions of Infections in Long-Term Care Facilities: Revisiting the McGeer Criteria. *Infect Cont Hosp Ep.* 2012; 33(10): 965–977.

[62] Ahmed A. Digoxin and reduction in mortality and hospitalization in geriatric heart failure: importance of low doses and low serum concentrations. *J Gerontol A Biol Sci Med Sci* 2007; 62(3):323–329.

[63] Nifedipine. Dose-related increase in mortality in patients with coronary heart disease. *Circulation* 1995; 92(5):1326–1331.

[64] Wyse DG, Waldo AL, DiMarco JP, et al. A comparison of rate control and rhythm control in patients with atrial fibrillation. *N Engl J Med.* 2002; 347:1825–1833.

[65] Carlsson J, Miketic S, Windeler J, et al. Randomized trial of rate-control versus rhythm-control in persistent atrial fibrillation: the Strategies of Treatment of Atrial Fibrillation (STAF) study. *J Am Coll Cardiol.* 2003; 41:1690–1696.

[66] Porter RS. (2011) The Merck Manual of Diagnosis and Therapy Nineteenth Edition.

[67] Fong TG, Tulebaev, SR, et al. Delirium in elderly adults: diagnosis, prevention and treatment. *Nat Rev Neurol.* 2009; 5(4):210–220.

[68] Coupland C, Dhiman P, Morriss R, Arthur A, Barton G and Hippisley-Cox J. Antidepressant use and risk of adverse outcomes in older people: population based cohort study. *BMJ* 2011; 343:d4551.

69 Coupland C, Dhiman P, et al. Antidepressant use and risk of adverse outcomes in older people: population based cohort study. *BMJ* 2011; 343:d4551.

70 Wooltorton E. Risperidone (Risperdal): increased rate of cerebrovascular events in dementia trials. *CMAJ* 2002; 167(11):1269–1270.

71 Maust DT, Kim HM, Seyfried LS et al. Antipsychotics, other psychotropics, and the risk of death in patients with dementia: number needed to harm. *JAMA Psychiatry*. 2015 May; 72(5):438–45.

72 Allain H, Bentue-Ferrer D, Polard E, et al. Postural instability and consequent falls and hip fractures associated with use of hypnotics in the elderly: a comparative review. *Drugs & Aging* 2005; 22(9):749–765.

73 Keston M, Brocklehurst JC. Flurazepam and meprobamate: a clinical trial. *Age & Ageing* 1974; 3(1):54–58.

74 Finkle WD, Der JS, Greenland S, et al. Risk of fractures requiring hospitalization after an initial prescription of zolpidem, alprazolam, lorazepam or diazepam in older adults. *J Am Geriatr Soc.* 2011; 59(10):1883–1890.

75 Cotroneo A, Gareri P, Nicoletti N, et al. Effectiveness and safety of hypnotic drugs in the treatment of insomnia in over 70-year old people. *Arch Gerontol Geriatr* 2007; 44(Suppl 1):121–124.

76 Hulley S, Grady D, Bush T, et al. Randomized trial of estrogen plus progestin for secondary prevention of coronary heart disease in postmenopausal women. *JAMA* 1998; 280: 605–613.

77 Writing Group for the Women's Health Initiative Investigators (2002). "Risks and Benefits of Estrogen Plus Progestin in Healthy Postmenopausal Women: Principal Results From the Women's Health Initiative Randomized Controlled Trial". *JAMA* 288(3): 321–333.

78 Hirsch IB. Sliding Scale Insulin—Time to Stop Sliding. *JAMA*. 2009 Jan 14; 301(2):213–4.

79 Lipska KJ, Ross JS, Wang Y, National Trends in US Hospital Admissions for Hyperglycemia and Hypoglycemia Among Medicare Beneficiaries, 1999 to 2011. *JAMA Intern Med.* 2014; 174(7):1116–1124.

80 ADOPT Kahn SE, Haffner SM, Heise MA, Herman WH, Holman RR, Jones NP, et al. Glycemic durability of rosiglitazone, metformin, or glyburide monotherapy. *N Engl J Med.* 2006; 355:2427–43.

81 DREAM Trial Investigators. Effect of rosiglitazone on the frequency of diabetes in patients with impaired glucose tolerance or impaired fasting glucose: a randomised controlled trial. *Lancet.* 2006; 368:1096–105.

82 Home PD, Pocock SJ, Beck-Nielsen H, Curtis PS, Gomis R, Hanefeld M, et al, RECORD Study Team. Rosiglitazone evaluated for cardiovascular outcomes in oral agent combination therapy for type 2 diabetes (RECORD): a multicentre, randomised, open-label trial. *Lancet.* 2009; 373:2125–35.

83 ACCORD Study Group. Effects of intensive glucose lowering in type 2 diabetes. *N Engl J Med.* 2008; 358:2545–59.

[84] Duckworth W, Abraira C, Moritz T, Reda D, Emanuele N, Reaven PD, et al: for the VADT Investigators. Glucose control and vascular complications in veterans with type 2 diabetes. *N Engl J Med.* 2009; 360:129–39.

[85] Shorr RI, Ray WA, Daugherty JR, et al. Individual sulfonylureas and serious hypoglycemia in older people. *J Am Geriatr Soc.* 1996; 44(7):751–755.

[86] Bateman DN, Rawlins MD, Simpson JM. Extrapyramidal reactions with metoclopramide. *Br Med J* (Clin Res Ed) 1985; 291(6500):930–932.

[87] Simmons A, Rouf E, Whittle, J. Not Your Typical Pneumonia: A Case of Exogenous Lipoid Pneumonia. *J Gen Intern Med* 22(11):1613–6.

[88] Durand C, Willett KC, Desilets AR. Proton Pump Inhibitor use in Hospitalized Patients: Is Overutilization Becoming a Problem? *Clin Med Insights Gastroenterol.* 2012; 5: 65–76.

[89] Kwok CS, Arthur AK, Anibueze CI. Risk of Clostridium difficile infection with acid suppressing drugs and antibiotics: meta-analysis. *Am J Gastroenterol.* 2012 Jul; 107(7):1011–9.

[90] CDC newsroom. Nearly half a million Americans suffered from Clostridium difficile infections in a single year. Feb 25, 2015. Retrieved from http://www.cdc.gov/media/releases/2015/p0225-clostridium-difficile.html Last accessed Dec 19, 2015.

[91] Gulmez SE, Holm A, Frederiksen H, et al. Use of proton pump inhibitors and the risk of community-acquired pneumonia: a population-based case-control study. *Arch Intern Med.* 2007; 167(9):950.

[92] McColl KE. Effect of proton pump inhibitors on vitamins and iron. *Am J Gastroenterol.* 2009; 104 Suppl 2:S5.

[93] Targownik LE, Lix LM, Metge CJ, et al. Use of proton pump inhibitors and risk of osteoporosis-related fractures. *CMAJ.* 2008; 179:319–326.

[94] Gomm W, von Holt K, Thome F, et al. Association of proton pump inhibitors with risk of dementia. *JAMA Neurol.* 2016 Feb 15. [Epub ahead of print].

[95] US FDA: Drug Safety and Availability. FDA Drug Safety Communication: FDA strengthens warning that non-aspirin nonsteroidal anti-inflammatory drugs (NSAIDs) can cause heart attacks or strokes Sept 9, 2015. http://www.fda.gov/Drugs/DrugSafety/ucm451800.htm. Last Acccessed Dec 19, 2015.

[96] Onder G, Pellicciotti F, Gambassi G, et al. NSAID-related psychiatric adverse events: who is at risk? *Drugs* 2004; 64(23):2619–2627.

[97] Billups SJ, Delate T, Hoover B. Injury in an elderly population before and after initiating a skeletal muscle relaxant. *Ann Pharmacother* 2011; 45(4):485–491.

[98] American Geriatrics Society 2015 Updated Beers Criteria for Potentially Inappropriate Medication Use in Older Adults. *J Am Geriatr Soc.* 2015; 63(11):2227–2246.

[99] Benca, RM. Diagnosis and Treatment of Chronic Insomnia: A Review. *Psychiatr Serv.* 2005 Mar; 56(3):332–43.

[100] Green GA. Understanding NSAIDs: from aspirin to COX-2. *Clin Cornerstone.* 2001; 3(5):50–60.

101 Adapted from: O'Mahony D, O'Sullivan D, Byrne S. STOPP/START criteria for potentially inappropriate prescribing in older people: version 2. *Age & Ageing*. 2015; 44(2): 213–218.

102 Feary JR, Rodrigues LC et al. Prevalence of major comorbidities in subjects with COPD and incidence of myocardial infarction and stroke: a comprehensive analysis using data from primary care. *Thorax* 2010; 65:956–962.

103 Lanas A, Wu P, et al. Low Doses of Acetylsalicylic Acid Increase Risk of Gastrointestinal Bleeding in a Meta-Analysis. *Clin Gastroenterol Hepatol* 2011; 9: 762–68.

104 Vandvik PO, Lincoff AM, Gore JM et al. Primary and secondary prevention of cardiovascular disease: Antithrombotic Therapy and Prevention of Thrombosis, 9th ed: American College of Chest Physicians Evidence-Based Clinical Practice Guidelines. *Chest*. 2012 Feb; 141(2 Suppl):e637S–68S.

105 Jacob S, Spinler, S. Hyponatremia Associated with Selective Serotonin-Reuptake Inhibitors in Older Adults. *Ann Pharmacother* 2006; 40:1618–22.

106 FDA Drug Safety Communication: FDA revises warnings regarding use of the diabetes medicine metformin in certain patients with reduced kidney function. http://www.fda.gov/Drugs/DrugSafety/ucm493244.htm. (Accessed April, 2016).

107 Brewer GJ. Iron and copper toxicity in diseases of aging, particularly atherosclerosis and Alzheimer's disease. *Exp Biol Med* (Maywood). 2007 Feb; 232(2):323–35.

108 World Health Organization. WHO's Pain Ladder. 1986. http://www.who.int/cancer/palliative/painladder/en/. Accessed May, 2016.

109 James PA, Oparil S, Carter BL et al. 2014 Evidence-Based Guideline for the Management of High Blood Pressure in Adults Report From the Panel Members Appointed to the Eighth Joint National Committee (JNC 8). [published erratum appears in *JAMA* 2014;311(17):1809] *JAMA*. 2014; 311(5):507–20.

110 Herrmann N, Lanctot K, Myszak M. Effectiveness of gabapentin for the treatment of behavioral disorders in dementia. *J Clin Psychopharmacol*. 2000; 20:90–93.

111 Influenza (Flu): Estimated Influenza Illnesses and Hospitalizations Averted by Vaccination — United States, 2014–15 Influenza Season. Dec 10, 2015. Accessed at: http://www.cdc.gov/flu/about/disease/2014–15.htm Last accessed Dec 20, 2015.

112 Thompson W, Shay D, Weintraub E et al. Mortality associated with influenza and respiratory syncytial virus in the United States. *JAMA* 2003; 289(2):179–86.

113 Dawood FS, Iuliano AD, Reed C, et al. Estimated global mortality associated with the first 12 months of 2009 pandemic influenza A H1N1 virus circulation: a modelling study. *The Lancet Infectious Diseases* 2012; (9):687–95.

114 Morbidity and Mortality Weekly Report (MMWR). Use of 13-Valent Pneumococcal Conjugate Vaccine and 23-Valent Pneumococcal Polysaccharide Vaccine Among Adults Aged ≥65 Years: Recommendations of the Advisory Committee on Immunization Practices (ACIP). Sept 19, 2014. Accessed online at: http://www.cdc.gov/mmwr/preview/mmwrhtml/mm6337a4.htm Last accessed Dec 20, 2015.

[115] Ten Medications Older Adults Should Avoid or Use with Caution. Adapted from: The American Geriatrics Society April 2012. Accessed online at: http://www.americangeriatrics. org/files/documents/beers/FHATipMEDS.pdf Last accessed Dec 20, 2015.

[116] Heatlh Information. Multivitamin/mineral Supplements Fact Sheet for Health Professionals. National Institutes of Health Office of Dietary Supplements. Accessed online at: http://ods. od.nih.gov/factsheets/MVMS-HealthProfessional/ Last accessed online on Dec 20, 2015.

[117] Bailey RL, Gahche JJ, Lentino CV, et al. Dietary supplement use in the United States, 2003–2006. *J Nutr.* 2011; 141(2):261–266.

[118] Folsom AR, Kushi LH, Anderson KE, et al. Associations of general and abdominal obesity with multiple health outcomes in older women: the Iowa Women's Health Study. *Arch Intern Med.* 2000;160(14):2117–2128.

[119] Guallar E, Stranges S, Mulrow S et al. Enough Is Enough: Stop Wasting Money on Vitamin and Mineral Supplements. *Ann Intern Med.* 2013;159:850–851.

[120] Sardar P, Chatterjee S, Chaudhari S et al. New Oral Anticoagulants in Elderly Adults: Evidence From a Meta-analysis of Randomized Trials. *J Am Geriatr Soc.* 2014; 62(5):857–864.

[121] Cranney C, Horsely T, O'Donnell S, et al. Effectiveness and safety of vitamin D. Evidence Report/Technology Assessment No. 158 prepared by the University of Ottawa Evidence-based Practice Center under Contract No. 290–02.0021. AHRQ Publication No. 07–E013. Rockville, MD: Agency for Healthcare Research and Quality, 2007.

[122] Gillespie WJ, Avenell A, Henry DA, et al. Vitamin D and vitamin D analogues for preventing fractures associated with involutional and post-menopausal osteoporosis (Cochrane Review) I. The Cochrane Library, issue 1. Update Software, Oxford. 2003.

[123] American Geriatrics Society Workgroup on Vitamin D Supplementation for Older Adults. Recommendations abstracted from the American Geriatrics Society Consensus Statement on vitamin D for Prevention of Falls and Their Consequences. *J Am Geriatr Soc.* 2014 Jan;62(1):147–52.

[124] Health Information. Vitamin D Fact Sheet for Health Professionals. National Institutes of Health Office of Dietary Supplements. Accessed online at: https://ods.od.nih.gov/ factsheets/VitaminD-HealthProfessional/ Last Accessed 12/20/2015.

[125] Grundman M. Vitamin E and Alzheimer disease: the basis for additional clinical trials. *Am J Clin Nutr.* 2000 Feb;71(2):630S–636S.

[126] Miller ER 3rd, Pastor-Barriuso R, Dalal D, et al. Meta-analysis: high-dosage vitamin E supplementation may increase all-cause mortality. *Ann Intern Med.* 2005;142(1):37.

[127] Sacks FM, Svetkey LP, Vollmer WM, et al. Effects on Blood Pressure of Reduced Dietary Sodium and the Dietary Approaches to Stop Hypertension (DASH) Diet. *N Engl J Med* 2001; 344:3–10.

[128] O'Donnell M, Mente A, Yusuf S. Hypertension Compendium: Sodium Intake and Cardiovascular Health. *Circulation Research.* 2015;116:1046–1057.

[129] Won AB, Lapane KL, Vallow S, et al. Persistent nonmalignant pain and analgesic prescribing patterns in elderly nursing home residents. *J Am Geriatr Soc.* 2004; 52:867.

[130] AGS Panel on Persistent Pain in Older Persons. The management of persistent pain in older persons. *J Am Geriatr Soc.* 2002; 50:S205.

[131] Shega JW, Dale W, Andrew M, et al. Persistent pain and frailty: a case for homeostenosis. *J Am Geriatr Soc.* 2012; 60:113.

[132] Weiner, D, Karp, J, Bernstein, C, et al. Pain Medicine in Older Adults: How Should it Differ? In: Comprehensive Treatment of Chronic Pain by Medical, Interventional and Behavioral Approaches. Deer, T, Ray, A, Gordin, V, et al. (Eds), Springer, 2012.

[133] Park J, Hughes AK. Nonpharmacological approaches to the management of chronic pain in community-dwelling older adults: a review of empirical evidence. *J Am Geriatr Soc.* 2012; 60:555.

[134] Kuehn BM. FDA focuses on drugs and liver damage: labeling and other changes for acetaminophen. *JAMA* 2009; 302:369.

[135] Scheiman JM, Hindley CE. Strategies to optimize treatment with NSAIDs in patients at risk for gastrointestinal and cardiovascular adverse events. *Clin Ther* 2010; 32:667.

[136] Coxib and traditional NSAID Trialists' (CNT) Collaboration, Bhala N, Emberson J, et al. Vascular and upper gastrointestinal effects of non-steroidal anti-inflammatory drugs: meta-analyses of individual participant data from randomised trials. *Lancet* 2013; 382:769.

[137] Coupland CA, Dhiman P, Barton G, et al. A study of the safety and harms of antidepressant drugs for older people: a cohort study using a large primary care database. *Health Technol Assess* 2011; 15:1.

[138] Coupland CA, Dhiman P, Barton G, et al. A study of the safety and harms of antidepressant drugs for older people: a cohort study using a large primary care database. *Health Technol Assess* 2011; 15:1.

[139] Reisner L. Pharmacological management of persistent pain in older persons. *J Pain* 2011; 12:S21.

[140] Moore RA, Straube S, Wiffen PJ, et al. Pregabalin for acute and chronic pain in adults. *Cochrane Database Syst Rev* 2009; CD007076.

[141] Straube S, Derry S, Moore RA, McQuay HJ. Pregabalin in fibromyalgia: meta-analysis of efficacy and safety from company clinical trial reports. *Rheumatology* (Oxford) 2010; 49:706.

[142] Reisner L. Pharmacological management of persistent pain in older persons. *J Pain* 2011; 12:S21.

[143] King S, Forbes K, Hanks GW, et al. A systematic review of the use of opioid medication for those with moderate to severe cancer pain and renal impairment: a European Palliative Care Research Collaborative opioid guidelines project. *Palliat Med* 2011; 25:525.

[144] Walsh SL, Preston KL, Stitzer ML, et al. Clinical pharmacology of buprenorphine: ceiling effects at high doses. *Clin Pharmacol Ther* 1994; 55:569.

[145] Stamer UM, Stüber F. Genetic factors in pain and its treatment. *Curr Opin Anaesthesiol* 2007; 20:478.

146 Kiely DK, Jons RN, Bergmann MA et al. Association between psychomotor activity delirium subtypes and mortality amongst newly admitted post-acute facility patients. *J Gerontol A Biol Sci Med Sci.* 2007;62(2):174–179.

147 Weiner DK, Hanlon JT, Studenski SA. Effects of central nervous system polypharmacy on falls liability in community-dwelling elderly. *Gerontology* 1998; 44:217.

148 McLachlan AJ, Bath S, Naganathan V, et al. Clinical pharmacology of analgesic medicines in older people: impact of frailty and cognitive impairment. *Br J Clin Pharmacol* 2011; 71:351.

149 Benedetti F, Arduino C, Costa S, et al. Loss of expectation-related mechanisms in Alzheimer's disease makes analgesic therapies less effective. *Pain* 2006; 121:133.

150 Chibnall JT, Tait RC, Harman B, Luebbert RA. Effect of acetaminophen on behavior, well-being, and psychotropic medication use in nursing home residents with moderate-to-severe dementia. *J Am Geriatr Soc* 2005; 53:1921.

151 Pharmacological Management of Persistent Pain in Older Persons (2009) http://www.centralhealthline.ca/healthlibrary_docs/painMgmt_for_Older_Persons.pdf (Accessed April 2016).

152 http://www.centralhealthline.ca/healthlibrary_docs/painMgmt_for_Older_Persons.pdf. Last accessed May 2016.

153 Mitchell SL, Teno JM, Kiely DK, et al. The clinical course of advanced dementia. *N Engl J Med* 2009; 361:1529.

154 Hanlon JT, Schmader KE, Samsa GP, et al. A method for assessing drug therapy appropriateness. *J Clin Epidemiol* 1992; 45:1045.

155 Steinman MA, Landefeld CS, Rosenthal GE, et al. Polypharmacy and prescribing quality in older people. *J Am Geriatr Soc* 2006; 54:1516.

156 Appel LJ, Espeland MA, Easter L, et al. Effects of reduced sodium intake on hypertension control in older individuals: results from the Trial of Nonpharmacologic Interventions in the Elderly (TONE). *Arch Intern Med* 2001; 161:685.

157 Advancing Adherence & the Science of Pharmacy Care. PQA/URAC Medication Adherence Summit. June 2011.

158 Alkema GE, Enguidanos SM, Wilber KH, et al. The role of consultant pharmacists in reducing medication problems among older adults receiving Medicaid waiver services. *Consult Pharm* 2009; 24:121–133.

159 Garfinkel D, Mangin D. Feasibility study of a systematic approach for discontinuation of multiple medications in older adults: Addressing polypharmacy. *Arch Intern Med* 2010; 170:1648.

160 Garfinkel D, Mangin D. Feasibility study of a systematic approach for discontinuation of multiple medications in older adults: addressing polypharmacy. *Arch Intern Med* 2010; 170:1648.

Made in the USA
Middletown, DE
13 May 2021